USMLE STEP 2 CK
Obstetrics & Gynecology
In Your Pocket

✓ Study guide for the USMLE STEP 2 CK exam.

✓ Prepare for your shelf examination.

✓ Be ready for your inpatient rotation.

Gregory J. Fernandez M.D.

First Edition, 2016
Author & Editor: Gregory J. Fernandez, M.D.
Publisher: M.D. Educational Services
Peer-reviewer: Joy Evans, MD
Book Design: Marie Meyer
Copyediting: Editage Cactus Communications

DISCLAIMER: The author, editor, publisher, and staff members have taken care to confirm the accuracy of the information present in this publication. The context of the books entirely, is believed to be reliable in accordance with the standards accepted at the time of publication. However, readers are encouraged to confirm the information and conduct their own research for clarification of all the information present within this book. No one involved in creating this book is responsible for errors or omissions or for any consequences from application of the information in this book. There is no warranty, expressed or implied, with respect to the completeness or accuracy of the contents of this publication. Neither the editor, nor the author assumes any liability for any injury and/or damage to persons or property arising from the content of this publication. Application of this information in a particular situation remains the professional responsibility of the practitioner; the clinical treatments or information described and recommended may not be considered absolute and universal recommendations. It is the responsibility of the health care provider to ascertain the FDA status of each drug used or device planned for use in their clinical practice. The purpose of this books, is to be used as a study guide for medical examinations. Please consult with attending physicians for any medical decisions.

ISBN-13: 978-1539969112

ISBN-10: 1539969118

This book is gratefully dedicated to my wife. Thank you for your support and always being there for me. Thank you for your kindness, your devotion, and your endless selflessness support. I love you… Thank you mother, father, step-mother, brothers, friends, and family for all your encouragement and endless love. Best of luck to all the medical dreamers, the road is long and I hope my book helps you through this journey. All the best…

How to Use

"Obstetrics & Gynecology In Your Pocket"

Gynecology In Your Pocket is a study guide for the USMLE STEP 2 CK exam that you can also use to prepare for your shelf examination and to get ready for your inpatient rotation. It is part of a series, each dealing with a different subject or sub-specialty, focusing on vital clinical knowledge.

The subjects and topics within gynecology are called out in large, colored type. These items are also included in the Table of Contents for ease of access.

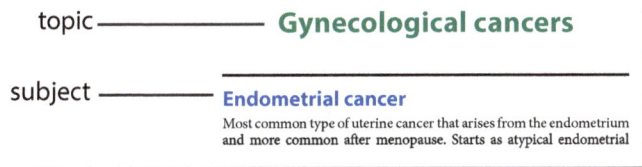

topic —————— **Gynecological cancers**

subject —————— **Endometrial cancer**
Most common type of uterine cancer that arises from the endometrium and more common after menopause. Starts as atypical endometrial

Many subjects also contain sub-subjects that are also called out in bold, blue type either as bulleted items or in-line with the text, as appropriate. They are all referenced in the index.

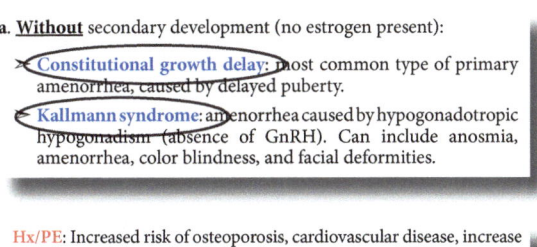

a. **Without** secondary development (no estrogen present):

> **Constitutional growth delay:** most common type of primary amenorrhea, caused by delayed puberty.
> **Kallmann syndrome:** amenorrhea caused by hypogonadotropic hypogonadism (absence of GnRH). Can include anosmia, amenorrhea, color blindness, and facial deformities.

Hx/PE: Increased risk of osteoporosis, cardiovascular disease, increase in LDL, mood change, hot flashes, dyspareunia, loss of libido, insomnia, vaginal dryness, and **vaginal atrophy** caused by low estrogen levels, which manifest as dyspareunia and vaginal bleeding after intercourse).

Presentation of clinical history and physical exam (Hx/PE), step-by-step diagnosis, and treatment plan are indicated by bold red headings.

be caused by follicular swelling of the ovarian wall. The pain can appear similar to appendicitis, menstrual cramps, or ovarian pathology.

Hx/PE: *Unilateral* pelvic pain (ovary rupture) mid-cycle.

Diagnosis: Pelvic examination (to rule out pathology), pelvic ultrasonography, and hCG level.

Treatment: NSAIDs (pain and inflammation) or OCPs (inhibit ovulation).

Note:

Procedures, triads, pathology, medications, antibodies and findings are called out in bold text. These items are also included in the index.

Treatment:
- If **small** (<3.5cm) and unruptured, give MTX.
- If **larger** (>3.5cm), consider **salpingectomy** (if ruptured) or **salpingostomy** (if not ruptured). These procedures cause risk of future ectopic pregnancies.
- Tubal rupture (obstetric emergency), will need laparoscopy/

Reflexes, signs and maneuvers are shown in purple text.

urinary or fecal incontinence, dyspareunia, and incomplete bladder emptying.

Diagnosis: Valsalva maneuver in lithotomy position.

Treatment:

Mnemonics and key words are shown in orange text.

- Rule out causes of amenorrhea with hCG, prolactin, TSH, and FSH/LH ratio.
- Pelvic ultrasonography (first step) "pearl necklace sign" may be visible.
- Increased total testosterone and DHEAS levels.
- 17-OH progesterone and 24-hour urine free cortisol (to rule

And, finally, for the avoidance of doubt, circumstances that amount to a medical emergency are flagged with a warning.

salpingostomy (if not ruptured). These procedures cause risk of future ectopic pregnancies.
- Tubal rupture (obstetric emergency) will need laparoscopy/ salpingectomy (removal of fallopian tube **plus** pregnancy).
- Give RhoGam to Rh-negative mother.

Obstetrics
Table of Contents

Gynecology
Table of Contents

Obstetrics

Obstetric terminology

Gravidity: number of times a patient has been pregnant.

Parity: number of pregnancies that led to birth beyond 20 weeks.

Naegele's rule = last menstrual periods (LMP) + 9 months + 7 days.

Developmental age: exact date of fertilization used for research.

Gestational age: can be determined by:

- LMP + 9 months + 7 days.
- Fundal height:
  - At 9 weeks, the fetus should be at the pelvis level.
  - At 20 weeks, the fetus should be at the umbilicus level.
- Quickening/movements → start at about 20 weeks.
- Fetal heart development → starts at about 10–12 weeks.
- Ultrasonography: most reliable during the first trimester to measure the **crown-rump length** at 5–12 weeks.
- After 13 weeks, measure femur length, biparietal diameter, or abdominal circumference.

Terms used for gestational age

➤ Abortion: <20 weeks.

➤ Intrauterine fetal demise: >20 weeks.

➤ Immature: <28 weeks.

➤ Pre-mature: <37 weeks.

➤ Mature: 37–42 weeks.

➤ Post-mature: >42 weeks.

Normal maternal physiological changes

➤ Increased GFR, renal blood flow, heart rate, cardiac output, systemic volume, respiratory rate, and alkaline phosphatase level.

➤ Decreased BUN/Cr ratio, blood pressure, peripheral vascular resistance, expiratory reserve, and sphincter tone.

Maternal calorie intake: increase intake to 100–300 kcal/day during pregnancy and 500 kcal/day when breastfeeding.

Recommended maternal weight gain

➤ Body mass index (BMI) <18.5 → mother should gain 28-40 Ibs during pregnancy.

➤ BMI (18.5–25) → gain 25-35 Ibs.

➤ BMI (25–30) → gain 15-25 Ibs.

➤ BMI (>30) → gain 11-20 Ibs.

➤ BMI (for twins)→ gain 35-45 Ibs.

Maternal supplementation

➤ Folic acid: give all women 0.4 mg/dL or 4.0 mg in cases of history of neurotube defects. Best to start supplementation at least 1 month before pregnancy.

- ➤ Iron: start at first visit 30 mg/day (elemental iron) or 150 mg/day (iron sulfate).
- ➤ Calcium: <19 years of age, give 1,300 mg/day and if >19 years of age, give 1,000 mg/day.
- ➤ Vitamin D: 10 µg/day.
- ➤ Vitamin B12: 2 µg/day.

Note: iron deficiency is the most common cause of anemia in pregnancy.

Normal neonatal growth

Newborn weight loss: newborns may lose up to 10% of the body weight in the first 10 days. Weight loss is partly caused by decreased bile production in neonates.

Normal children's weight gain: weight doubles by 6 months, triples by 1 year, and quadruples by 2 years ("6, 1, 2").

Normal children's length gain: length increases by ½ by 1 year, doubles by 4 years, and triples by puberty ("1, 4, 13").

Normal maternal exercise: 30 minutes/day of mild to moderate exercise is recommended.

Maternal screening

Maternal initial visit laboratory studies

Initial visit order and measure: blood pressure, CBC (<10 g/dL is considered anemia), electrolytes, hepatitis B and C, HIV (need consent for HIV testing), PPD, VDRL, rubella antibody, Pap smear, G&C, fasting glucose, type and screening, Rh factor, urinalysis, and urine culture.

Note: asymptomatic UTIs during pregnancy (no symptoms with positive urinalysis) will need to be treated.

Maternal screening:

- 9–14 weeks: **pregnancy-associated plasma protein A (PAPP-A)** plus nuchal translucency ultrasound plus B-HCG. +/- chorionic villus sampling (CVS).
- 15–20 weeks: amniocentesis if quad-screening is abnormal or if there are other indications for amniocentesis.
- 18–20 weeks: ultrasonography for anatomic screening.
- 24–28 weeks: 1-hour glucose challenge test.
- 28–30 weeks: give RhoGAM to all Rh-negative patients.
- 32–36 weeks: CBC and GBS culture.
- 34–40 weeks: Pap smear and HIV/ RPR for high-risk patients.

Maternal scheduled visits

- 0–28 weeks: visit every month.
- 29–35 weeks: visit every 2 weeks.
- 36 weeks–birth: visit every week.

Human chorionic gonadotropin (hCG)

- Urine hCG (sensitive) or serum hCG (specific): standard diagnosis for pregnancy.
- First test ordered for all patients with amenorrhea.
- Produced in the placenta and peaks at 100,000 mlU/ml at 10 weeks.
- Doubles every 48 hours during the first trimester and can be used to rule out ectopic pregnancy and choriocarcinoma.
- hCG maintains the corpus luteum.

Quadruple screening

Measuring β-HCG, inhibin A, AFP, and unconjugated estriol levels.

- Increased MS-AFP: (>2.5 MoMs). Produced by the fetus.

- Associated with incorrect gestation dating (most commonly), open neural tube defects, anencephaly, spina bifida, gastroschisis, omphalocele, and multiple gestations.
- Spina bifida needs surgery within 24-48 hours after delivery.

Note: elevated MS-AFP necessitates repeat ultrasonography to confirm gestational dates. Keep in mind that an early gestational ultrasonography is more accurate.

- Decreased MS-AFP: (< 0.5 MoMs).
  - Associated with trisomy 21 and 18, fetal demise, and inaccurate dating.

Diagnosis:
- In cases of low or elevated MS-AFP the next step would be obstetric ultrasonography to confirm gestation date.
- If the dates are accurate the next step would be amniocentesis or CVS and AF-AFP measurement.

Down syndrome

Quadruple screening: increased β-HCG and inhibin A levels and decreased AFP and unconjugated estriol levels.

Note: adolescent pregnancies does not increase the risk of Down's syndrome.

Edward's syndrome

Quadruple screening: decreased β-HCG, inhibin A, AFP, and unconjugated estriol levels

---

Pregnancy-associated plasma protein A (PAPP-A)

Measured between 9 and 14 weeks. The benefit is that less invasive than CVS.

Ultrasound-determined nuchal translucency <u>plus</u> β-hCG can detect 85% of Down's syndrome and 97% of Edward's syndrome cases.

Chorionic villus sampling (CVS)

Procedure can be done between 9 and 13 weeks.

Used for early genetic screening (such as Down's syndrome) and can be performed via transcervical or transabdominal aspiration.

<u>Disadvantages</u>: fetal loss, infection, hemorrhage, and inability to detect neural tube defects.

Note: CVS done <9 weeks can be associated with limb defects.

Amniocentesis

Procedure can be done between 15 and 20 weeks.

Genetic screening via transabdominal aspiration with ultrasound-guided needle.

- ➤ <u>Advantage</u>: can detect open neural tube defects.
- ➤ <u>Disadvantages</u>: premature rupture of membrane (PROM), infection, and hemorrhage.

<u>Indications</u>: >35 years of age, abnormal quadruple screening with confirmed fetal dating, or history of genetic diseases. Can be used to measure lecithin to sphingomyelin ratio. Need to give Rh-negative mothers RhoGAM before procedure.

Note: screening for advanced paternal age is not routinely recommended.

RhoGAM

- 300mcg prophylactic dose is given at 28 weeks of gestation and again <u>after</u> delivery.
- Administered when there is increased risk of hemorrhage, abortion, ectopic pregnancy, amniocentesis, CVS, or trauma.

- The fetus is at risk in Rh-negative mothers, not Rh-positive mothers.
- If fetomaternal hemorrhage is suspected, perform a **Rosette test.**

Category X medications

Medications in pregnancy that are absolute contraindications.

- ➤ Isotretinoin: cleft lip/palate and thymic aplasia.
- ➤ Warfarin: epiphyses striping and nasal hypoplasia.
- ➤ Thalidomide: bilateral limb defects.

Category C medications

- ➤ Means animal studies have shown fetal risk, but no human studies have yet been conducted.

Maternal screening: "TORCHES" infections

Toxoplasmosis

In pregnant women can be caused by raw meat or cat feces. Educate mothers about risks.

Hx/PE: Causes intracranial calcifications, microcephaly, hydrocephalus, and failure to thrive in neonates.

Diagnosis:

- *Best initial test*: head CT scan (*multiple* hypodense "ring-enhancing lesions").
- Serologic testing with PCR (*most accurate*).
- Repeat head CT scan after treatment.

Treatment: Pyrimethamine + sulfadiazine + folic acid.

Prevention: educate mothers about avoiding handling the litter box and raw meats during the first trimester.

Rubella

Rubella (ss-RNA from the *Togaviridae* family) virus causes "blueberry muffin" rash, cataract, hearing loss, mental retardation, and PDA.

Diagnosis: Serologic testing with PCR and maternal screening during first office visit.

Treatment:

- Supportive care (fluids, NSAIDs, and rest). No post-exposure prophylaxis available.
- Screen with ophthalmic examination, echocardiogram, and hearing test.

Prevention: vaccination with MMR before pregnancy (recommended at least 1 month prior but not during pregnancy). No real evidence against side effects but has become the standard.

CMV

Most common congenital viral infection in the United States. Transmitted transplacentally (body fluid secretions) and can cause periventricular calcifications with microcephaly, deafness, pneumonia, and jaundice.

Diagnosis: *Best initial test* is urine or saliva viral titer (most accurate is urine or saliva PCR).

Treatment: Post-partum ganciclovir or foscarnet (treatment prevents viral shedding but does not treat infection).

Herpes virus

Can effect multiple locations including the skin, eyes, CNS, and systemic system. Neonates have a 50% morality rate and survivors can develop mental retardation and meningoencephalitis.

Diagnosis:

- Clinical diagnosis (no other tests needed).
- *Best initial test*: serologic testing with **Tzanck smear** (if needed).
- *Most specific test*: HSV PCR.

Treatment:

- If lesions are present at term, give mother oral acyclovir and deliver via C-section.
- Start prophylaxis in pregnant women at 36 weeks in case of history of herpes.
- Avoid fetal scalp electrodes, as these can transmit HSV to the neonate.

Human immunodeficiency virus (HIV)

Need to avoid invasive procedures. Can be transmitted in utero, during delivery, or via breast milk.

Diagnosis:

- Women have the right to refuse HIV testing but should be highly encouraged.
  - Need consent for testing patients for HIV.
- ELISA test (*sensitive*) and Western blot (*specific*).
- Test results can be false-positive (passive transport from mothers [IgG]). Results can be positive for newborns for up to 12-18 months of age.
  - If positive results are obtained during this time, it does not mean they have the disease.

Treatment:

- Start anti-retroviral therapy in all pregnant patients with combination therapy as early as possible plus start neonate on AZT therapy for 6 weeks postpartum.
- C-section if viral load >1,000 cells/mm3.
  - Elevated viral load is the biggest risk factor for transmission.
  - Low CDD+4 is not as much of a risk factor.
- Mothers with HIV should not breastfeed.

Note: triple therapy (most important method for risk factor prevention) along with cesarean delivery can decrease the transmission risk to only 2%.

Syphilis

Hx/PE: **Late-acquired congenital syphilis** (diagnosed usually after 2 years of age); symptoms include saddle nose, saber shins, peg-shaped upper incisors, deafness, and **Hutchinson's triad**.

Diagnosis:

- *Best initial test* is VDRL/RPR (screening) or Dark-field (1° disease) and FTA-ABS (2° and 3° disease) are the most accurate.
- Mothers with one STD need to be screened for other STDs.
- If screening test (VDRL) results are normal, confirm with FTA-ABS (*specific*).

Treatment: IM Penicillin G.

Note: if allergic to penicillin, desensitize the patient.

Obstetric examination

First stage labor: pre-delivery of neonate

- **Latent stage**: cervical dilation of <3 cm. Arrest can be caused by excessive sedation or hypotonic uterine contraction. Keep in mind that in the latent stage, there might not be any physical changes for hours. This does not always mean arrest of labor.

  ➤ Prolonged latent stage is >20 hours for primipara.

  ➤ Prolonged latent stage is >14 hour for multipara.

  Treatment: Decrease analgesics.

- **Active stage**: >4–10 cm dilation. Arrest caused by cephalopelvic disproportion.

- ➤ Prolonged active stage is <1.2 cm/hour of cervical dilation (primipara).
- ➤ Prolonged active state is <1.5 cm/hour of cervical dilation (multipara).
- ➤ No dilation in 2 hours is considered arrest.

Treatment:

- In case of *adequate* contractions, consider C-section.
- In case of *hypertonic* contractions, consider IV morphine.
- In case of *hypotonic* contractions, consider IV oxytocin.

Second stage labor: delivery of infant

- Prolonged if >2 hours in primipara.
- Prolonged if >1 hour in multipara.
- Can add an extra hour in case of epidural use.

  Treatment: Decrease epidural rate, start oxytocin, assisted vaginal delivery (forceps or vacuum), or C-section.

  Note: oxytocin (ADH-like hormone) can cause water retention and hyponatremia.

Third stage labor: delivery of placenta

- Prolonged if >30 minutes.

Treatment:

- If prolonged, consider oxytocin infusion (*first*) and manual removal (if oxytocin fails).
- Hysterectomy is rarely needed.

Leopold's maneuvers: manual determination of fetal position (longitudinal, oblique, or transverse).

Cervical examination:

   i.   Dilation.

   ii. Effacement.

   iii. Station.

   iv. Position.

   v. Consistency.

Note: there is <u>no</u> increased risk of abortions with retroverted uterus.

Bishop score

Favorability of delivery. Based on cervical examination. Total number of 15 points possible.

- ➢ <u>Score 10–15</u>: no intervention needed.
- ➢ <u>Score 5–9</u>: give Pitocin for induction.
- ➢ <u>Score 0–4</u>: C-section.

Rupture of membrane: requires sterile speculum examination.

Monitoring fetal heart rate

Most common obstetric procedure. Electrode attached to the fetal scalp (more precise) or Doppler ultrasonography (less invasive).

- ▪ Tachycardia: >160 (hypoxia and/or fetal anemia).
- ▪ Bradycardia: <110 (severe hypoxia and/or cord compressions).

- ➢ **Normal variability**: 6–25 bpm from beat to beat.
- ➢ **Minimal variability**: <6 bpm.
- ➢ **Marked variability**: >25 bpm.
- ➢ **Sinusoidal variability**: severe fetal anemia or narcotics given to mother.

Fetal heart rate decelerations

➤ **Early** **fetal heart rate decelerations**: normal findings that are caused by head compression.

➤ **Late** **fetal heart rate decelerations**: caused by uteroplacental insufficiency (including placental abruption), fetal distress, and hypoxia.

➤ **Variable** **fetal heart rate decelerations** (*most concerning*): cord compression.

Treatment: *First step* in management for variable decelerations will be to change maternal position and give oxygen.

Fetal heart rate accelerations: is reassuring and shows ability to respond to environment.

Fetal surveillance

➤ Fetal heart rate monitoring (*without* complications):

- First stage: measure every 30 minutes.
- Second stage: measure every 15 minutes.

➤ Fetal heart rate monitoring (with complications):

- First stage: measure every 15 minutes.
- Second stage: measure every 5 minutes.

Fetal movement assessment: normal fetal movements is about 10 movements over 20 minutes. If there are fewer than 10 movements, then conduct non-stress test (NST).

Non-stress test (NST)

Place mother in lateral tilt position with external measurement performed by Doppler ultrasonography.

➤ **Reactive NST** (*normal*): at least 2 accelerations, >15 bpm, >15 seconds; over 20 minutes.

➤ **Non-reactive NST** (*abnormal*): <2 accelerations, <15 bpm, <15 seconds; over 20 minutes.

Causes of positive non-reactive NST: sleeping fetus, maternal narcotic use, or fetal CNS abnormalities.

If non-reactive test results are positive, perform stress test or biophysical profile (BPP).

Stress tests

➤ **Contraction stress test (CST)**: mother in lateral position with nipple stimulation or oxytocin administration.

- **Positive** CST (*abnormal*): <u>late</u> deceleration in 50% of the contractions in 10 minutes. (Positive = fetal compromise and possible delivery).

- **Negative** CST (*normal*): late or variable deceleration <50% within 10 minutes.

Note: test contraindications are placenta previa, preterm membrane rupture, or high-risk preterm labor.

➤ **Biophysical profile** (BPP)

Real-time ultrasonography. "Test baby MAN" each worth (0–2 points): Tone, breathing, movement, amniotic fluid volume, and NST.

- Range 8–10: fetus is healthy; repeat test in 1–2 weeks.

- Range 4–6: is worrisome and if fetus is >36 weeks, then deliver. If <36 weeks, repeat in 12–24 hours.

- Range 0–3: indicates fetal hypoxia; immediate delivery required despite gestational age.

Modified biophysical profile (MBP)

NST and amniotic fluid level measured by ultrasonography (in 4 quadrants). Normal in case of reactive NST and amniotic fluid index (AFI) >5 cm.

Umbilical artery Doppler velocimetry

Used in intrauterine growth restriction (IUGR), to monitor reduction of blood flow.

Analgesia during pregnancy

Can decrease uterine contractions and cervical dilation.

<u>Types</u>:

➤ Local lidocaine (episiotomy).

➤ Epidural (*most effective*).

➤ Spinal (rapid onset and short duration).

<u>Side effects</u>: can cause constipation, decreased contractions, and aspiration pneumonia (secondary to delayed gag reflex and delayed gastric emptying). Will need prophylaxis PPIs to prevent aspiration.

<u>Contraindications</u>: maternal hypotension, coagulopathy, maternal bacteremia, skin infection over the site of needle placement, and increased cerebral pressure caused by mass lesion.

Teratogenic agents

➤ <u>ACEIs</u>: renal tubular dysplasia, oligohydramnios, and IUGR.

➤ <u>Alcohol</u>: **fetal alcohol syndrome** (midface hypoplasia, microcephaly, long philtrum, VSD, mental retardation; increased risk with >6 drinks/day).

➤ <u>Androgens</u>:
  - Females: virilization.
  - Males: advanced genital development.

➤ <u>Carbamazepine</u>: neural tube defects, fingernail hypoplasia, microcephaly, and IUGR.

➤ <u>Cocaine</u>: spontaneous abortion, bowel atresia, malformation of the heart, limbs, and face. GU and IUGR. Symptoms: high-pitched cries, irritability, tachypnea, tremors, and excessive sucking.

- DES: **clear cell adenocarcinoma** of the vagina or cervix. Risk of ectopic pregnancies.
- Lead: stillbirth and spontaneous abortion.
- Lithium: **Ebstein's anomaly** (tricuspid valve in the right ventricle).
- Methotrexate (MTX): spontaneous abortion.
- Mercury: mental retardation, seizure, microcephaly, and cerebral atrophy.
- Phenytoin: **fetal hydantoin**, fingernail hypoplasia, digit hypoplasia, cleft lip and palate, microcephaly, and mental retardation.
- Radiation: maximum dosage is 5 rads. Risk of microcephaly and mental retardation.
- Streptomycin: hearing loss and CN VIII damage (ototoxicity).
- Tetracycline: yellow-brown discoloration of the teeth and hypoplasia of the tooth enamel.
- Thalidomide: bilateral limb deficiencies.
- Valproic acid: neural tube defects, spina bifida, risk of cleft lip, meningomyelocele, craniofacial anomalies, long philtrum, high forehead, and small mouth.
- Vitamin A: hydrocephalus, microcephaly, thymic agenesis, cleft lip and cleft palate, and microphthalmia.
- Warfarin: stippled bone epiphyses, nasal hypoplasia, and ophthalmologic abnormalities.
- Opiates: hyperirritability, yawning, sneezing, distress, tremors, and diarrhea.

Oral contraceptives (combined estrogen and progesterone)

- Contraindications are pulmonary embolism, DVT, MI, strokes, SLE, smoking with age >35 years, unexplained uterine bleeding, pregnancy, and liver disease.

- Stop OCPs one month before desired pregnancy and start folic acid at 0.4 mg/day (if no risk factors). Higher dose of folic acid required if risk factors present.
- If a woman on OCPs becomes pregnant and in the first trimester, there is no risk of fetal malformations.
- Those on levothyroxine will need to increase dosage while on OCPs (remember that estrogen increases TBG).
- As opposed to OCPs, implantable or injectable contraceptives are associated with a lower pregnancy rate. OCPs can be used inconsistently and incorrectly, making them less effective.
- OCPs are <u>not</u> as effective as IUDs.
- Anti-seizure medications can decrease OCP efficacy.
- There is no association between combination OCP use and weight gain.
- **Ulipristal** is the most effective oral emergency contraception.
- OCPs decrease the risk of ovarian cancer.

Abortions

Spontaneous abortion

- Occurs <u>before</u> the 20th week of pregnancy, where 80% occur in the first trimester.
- 50% are caused by chromosomal abnormalities in the first trimester.
- 25% of all pregnancies end in elective abortion.

Risk factors: increased maternal age, infection, dietary deficiencies, inherited thrombophilia's (factor V, proteins C and S, and hyperhomocysteinemia), antiphospholipid antibodies, incompetent cervix, cervical injury, anatomical abnormalities of the cervix, diabetes, thyroid dysfunction, alcohol consumption, caffeine consumption, drug use, and radiation.

Diagnosis: Physical examination, CBC, serum hCG level (low), abdominal ultrasonography (can identify gestational sac at 5–6 weeks from LMP), fetal monitoring, Rh factor blood test, and urine toxicology testing, if suspicious.

Treatment:

- Treatment will depend on trimester and the type of abortion. *See below.
- Give RhoGAM, if mother is Rh-negative.

Complete abortion

Hx/PE: Product is completely expelled with the cervix closed.

Diagnosis:

- Pelvic ultrasound (empty uterus and no FHR).
- Need to monitor β-human chorionic gonadotropin (β-hCG) levels to ensure return to baseline levels.

Treatment: Refer patient for psychiatric support.

Note: helpful to rule out urine toxicology for abortions.

Incomplete abortion

Hx/PE: Presents with uterine bleeding and some product with opened os.

Diagnosis:

- Pelvic ultrasound (retained fetal tissue with no FHR).
- Need to ensure hCG levels return to baseline after treatment.

Treatment:

- Manual uterine aspiration (MUA) <u>or</u> dilation and curettage (D&C) if <13 weeks.
- Give RhoGAM, if mother is Rh-negative.
- Psychiatric support.

Threatened abortion

Hx/PE: Uterine bleeding, retained products, and closed os.

Diagnosis: Pelvic ultrasound (intact product and FHR present).

Treatment:

- Pelvic rest for 24–48 hours and no sexual intercourse.
- Give RhoGAM, if mother is Rh-negative.

Inevitable abortion

Hx/PE: Uterine bleeding, open os, and no product expelled.

Diagnosis:

- Pelvic ultrasound shows FHR and fetal tissue.
- Physical examination (retained open os +/-ROM).

Treatment:

- Product might evacuate spontaneously or use MUA or D&C (<13 weeks).
- Give RhoGAM, if mother is Rh-negative.
- Psychiatric support.

Missed abortion

Hx/PE: Product present, FHR absent, uterine bleeding absent, and closed os.

Diagnosis:

- Pelvic ultrasound: product present and FHR absent.
- Need to monitor hCG levels to ensure it returns to baseline.

Treatment: Depends on gestational age (MUA, D&C, or D&E). Psychiatric support.

Note: as a rule of thumb, in the first trimester perform D&C and in the second trimester perform dilation and evacuation (D&E).

Intrauterine fetal demise

Also known as stillbirth; defined as absence of fetal cardiac activity and no fetal movements after 20 weeks.

Diagnosis: Pelvic ultrasonography (no fetal heart tracing and inactive fetus).

Treatment: Induce labor or D&E. Removing the fetus, decreases the risk of DIC.

Note:

- ✓ Patient will need scheduled induction of labor, with the hope of obtaining an intact fetus for autopsy.
- ✓ D&E can be done but this will destroy the fetus, making the autopsy difficult.

Elective abortions

About 25% of all pregnancies in the United States end with elective abortions. Physicians have the right not to participate in abortions but need to refer patients to physicians that will.

➢ First trimester (first 3 months):

- Medications: oral mifepristone (RU486) + oral/vaginal misoprostol or another combination MTX + oral/vaginal misoprostol.
- Surgical: MUA or D&C with gentle aspiration.

➢ Second trimester: prostaglandins, oxytocin, and surgical D&E.

Levonorgestrel: emergency contraceptive that is sold over the counter for women aged >18 years. Is effective up to 5 days.

Premature rupture of membrane (PROM)

Rupture of the fetal membrane before onset of labor. Most common risk of PROM is ascending infections (chorioamnionitis). Rupture of membrane at <37 weeks.

Hx/PE: Gush of clear or blood-tinged amniotic fluid, <u>w/o</u> uterine contractions. Women in the third trimester have urine loss, so this needs to be ruled out.

Diagnosis:

- <u>First step</u>: pelvic ultrasonography (monitor amniotic fluid volume, fetal position, and fetal heart). Need to rule out placenta previa, as speculum examination could be dangerous in this case.
- <u>Second step</u>: **sterile speculum examination** (pooling of amniotic fluid).
  - **Nitrazine paper test** (positive if turns blue; alkaline amniotic fluid).
  - **Fern test** (ferning pattern seen under the microscope).
  - If unsure, use transabdominal instillation of **indigo carmine dye** (help visualize leaks).
- <u>Rule out chorioamnionitis</u>: leukocytosis, fever, and uterine tenderness.
- Always check CBC, PT/INR, PTT, bleeding time, platelets, blood type, Rh antibody screen, GBS status, fetal presentation, and fetal lung maturity.

Note: no digital vaginal examination if not in labor or labor not planned immediately (as this can induce infection).

Treatment: **Depends on gestational age and fetal lung maturity:**

- <u>If <32 weeks</u>: treat with bed rest, pelvic rest, prophylactic antibiotics, RhoGAM (if needed), and betamethasone 2 doses spaced within 12 hours apart to promote fetal lung maturity.
- <u>If >37 weeks:</u> labor induction with oxytocin can be considered (need to consider fetal presentation and fetal well-being).
- <u>If patients develop chorioamnionitis</u>, start IV antibiotics.
- RhoGAM given if mother is Rh-negative.

Note: GBS prophylaxis: if allergic to penicillin or amoxicillin then use clindamycin.

Preterm labor

Considered preterm at 28–37 weeks of gestation. Primary cause of neonatal morbidity and mortality.

Risk factors: many causes including, trauma, multiple gestation, infection, PROM, polyhydramnios, low SES, poor maternal nutrition, and cervical insufficiency.

Hx/PE: Pelvic pressure, low back pain, contractions, vaginal bleeding, and menstruation-like cramps.

Diagnosis:

- **True labor**: uterine contractions (≥3 contractions, lasting 30 seconds, over 30 minutes [is considered normal]) and cervical changes.
- Pelvic ultrasonography: monitor gestational age, fetal heart rate, fetal or uterine abnormalities, fetal presentation, and amniotic fluid volume.
- Culture for chlamydia, gonorrhea, and GBS.

Contraindications to tocolytic therapy: infection, non-reassuring fetal testing, and placental abruption.

Treatment:

- Bed rest, pelvic rest, tocolytics, steroids (IM), and penicillin or ampicillin for GBS prophylaxis (if preterm delivery is likely), preferably given 4 hours prior to delivery.
- History of **cervical incompetence**: place pessary at 12 weeks and remove at 36–38 weeks. Patients must not engage in sexual intercourse, heavy lifting, or prolonged standing during this time.

Note: antenatal corticosteroid therapy is given IM not IV.

Complications of prematurity: respiratory distress syndrome (RDS), PDA, necrotizing enterocolitis, inguinal hernias, and death.

Medical complications of pregnancy

Hyperemesis gravidarum

Caused by elevated levels of β-hCG and estradiol. Can be associated with multiple gestations and molar pregnancy. If morning sickness persists after the first trimester, consider hyperemesis gravidarum.

Hx/PE: Persistent nausea, vomiting, and dehydration.

Diagnosis:

- Serum hCG levels and ultrasonography to rule out molar pregnancy or multiple gestation.
- ABG (metabolic alkalosis) and electrolytes (hyponatremia, hypokalemia, and hypochloremia).

Treatment:

- *Mild cases*: first step is supplementation with vitamin B6, ginger lollipops, saltine crackers, small frequent meals, and tea.
- *Moderate cases*: doxylamine (anti-histamine) or promethazine (anti-histamine).
- *Severe cases*: metoclopramide (dopamine antagonist) or ondansetron (serotonin antagonist).
- *Severe dehydration*: administer IV fluids and dimenhydrinate.

Diabetes in pregnancy

Types:

➤ **Pregestational diabetes** (diagnosed before pregnancy).

➤ **Gestational diabetes** (diagnosed during pregnancy).

Pregestational diabetes

Hx/PE:

> *Maternal complications*: retinopathy, nephropathy, and neuropathy.

> *Fetus complications*: macrosomia, transposition of the great vessels, and hypoglycemia.

Note: congenital malformations are strongly associated with an HbA1c level >8.5 during the first trimester.

Diagnosis:

- Screening for pregestational diabetes is conducted by measuring the fasting glucose level during the first office visit (optimal fasting glucose < 95 mg/dL).
- Two positive test results <u>before</u> the 20 week of gestation indicates pregestational diabetes.
- Monitor fetus by ultrasonography (monthly), HbA1c (every 3 months), echocardiogram (start at 24 weeks), and NST (at 32 weeks), and induce labor at 39–40 weeks.
  - Ultrasonography required every month to assess fetal macrosomia or IUGR.

<u>Prevention for mother</u>: ophthalmic examination, renal examination (microalbuminuria), and foot examination.

Treatment:

- ADA diet, light exercise, and frequent home glucose monitoring.
- If not controlled by diet and exercise, start insulin (treatment of choice).
- Glucose goals: fasting glucose level <95 mg/dL and 1 hour postprandial glucose level <120 mg/dL.

Fun facts:

✓ During delivery, the goal is to control glucose levels between 80 and 100 mg/dL with IV insulin, 5% dextrose, and normal saline.

✓ Check glucose levels every 2 hours in the latent stage of labor and every hour during the active stage.

✓ After delivery, discontinue IV insulin.

✓ Early delivery is recommended if develop preeclampsia, macrosomia, or fetal lung maturity.

✓ Target gestational age for delivery is between 39 to 40 weeks.

✓ Cesarean delivery required if fetal weight is >4,500g (4.5 kg).

Gestational diabetes

Observed in 3–10% of all pregnancies and 50% of these patients develop diabetes mellitus postpartum. Glucose intolerance at any time postpartum is considered diabetes mellitus.

Hx/PE:

➤ *Maternal risks*: polyhydramnios, postpartum hemorrhage, mortality, cephalopelvic disproportion, preeclampsia, eclampsia, fetus large for gestational age, and edema.

➤ *Fetus risks*: hypocalcemia, hypomagnesemia, hypoglycemia (always check neonatal blood glucose levels), RDS, hyperbilirubinemia, IUGR, shoulder dystocia defects, small left colon, meconium plugging, cardiac anomalies (hypertrophic interventricular septum), and renal abnormalities.

Diagnosis:

- Diagnosed during the 24–28-week glucose screening test:

  - Start screening with a 1 hour **50g glucose challenge test** (drink within 5 min):

    - Fasting glucose level should be less than 95 mg/dL.

    - 1 hour level of >140 mg/dL is abnormal.

  - If abnormal, confirmatory test is with 3 hour **100g glucose challenge test**:

    - Fasting (>95 mg/dL), at 1 hour (>180 mg/dL), at 2 hours (>155 mg/dL), at 3 hours (>140 mg/dL).

    - 1 abnormal value indicates **impaired glucose tolerance**.

    - 2 abnormal values indicates gestational diabetes.

- Monitor fetus by ultrasonography (monthly), HbA1c (every 3 months), echocardiogram (start at 24 weeks), and NST (at 32 weeks), and induce labor at 39–40 weeks.

- During labor, check glucose levels every 2 hours in the latent stage and every 1 hour in the active stage.

Treatment:

- *First*: ADA diet (most important), light exercise, and glucose monitoring 4 times a day.
- *Second*: add insulin, if dietary control is insufficient.

Note:

- ✓ During pregnancy use insulin lispro and avoid using glargine.
- ✓ Perform a 2 hour 75g OGTT at 3 months after delivery to check if the diabetes has resolved.

Chronic hypertension

Blood pressure >140/90 mmHg, diagnosed before conception or before 20 weeks of gestation.

If a woman is diagnosed with hypertension before 20 weeks of gestation and presents with proteinuria after 20 weeks, the condition is referred to as **preeclampsia on chronic hypertension**.

Diagnosis:

- Measure blood pressure at every office visit.
- If the patient is diagnosed with hypertension before 20 weeks, then the condition is termed as chronic hypertension.
- Perform a urine dipstick and urinalysis (observe for proteins to rule out preeclampsia).

Treatment:

- *Stage 1* or mild hypertension (140-160/90-100 mmHg), treatment is not required.
- *Stage 2* hypertension (160-180/100-110 mmHg), medication choices are labetalol, hydralazine, methyldopa, and calcium channel blockers (*second line medications*).
- Anti-diuretics are not recommended (thiazides, loops diuretics, and ACEIs).

- Patients diagnosed with Raynaud's syndrome and well controlled on calcium channel blockers can continue medication.

Note: diuretics are contraindicated during pregnancy.

Gestational hypertension

Diagnosed <u>after</u> 20 weeks of gestation and usually returns to baseline by about 6 weeks postpartum. May progress to preeclampsia or eclampsia.

Diagnosis:

- Measure blood pressure at every office visit.
- If abnormal, perform urinalysis and urine dipstick test.

Treatment: Start treatment at *stage 2* hypertension (>160/100 mmHg) with labetalol, hydralazine, or methyldopa.

Note: anti-hypertensive medications can decrease blood flow to the placenta.

Mild preeclampsia

New-onset hypertension diagnosed <u>after</u> >20 weeks of gestation. Blood pressure >140/90 on 2 separate occasions; proteinuria >300mg in 24 hours or urine dipstick (+1-2 positive).

Hx/PE: Women with previous preeclampsia have a higher risk of preeclampsia in future pregnancies. Patients present with hypertension, proteinuria, and mild edema.

Diagnosis:

- Blood pressure measurement, urinalysis, urine dipstick, and 24-hour urine protein test.
- Need to rule out HELLP syndrome: CBC (anemia/platelets) and LFTs.

Treatment:

- *Preterm fetus* and if mother is stable: bed rest and monitor in hospital if the fetus is <u>less</u> than 34 weeks and if newly diagnosed case.

- *Term or worsening*: induce labor with IV oxytocin, prostaglandin, or amniotomy.
- Delivery by C-section or labor induction is curative.

Note: patient needs to be monitored and hospitalized, as the condition can rapidly progress to severe eclampsia.

Severe preeclampsia

Diagnosed <u>after</u> >20 weeks of gestation; blood pressure >160/100 mmHg on two occasions, >5 g protein in 24-hour urine protein test or +3-4 positive in urine dipstick.

Hx/PE: Similar symptoms as hypertension: headaches, blurred vision, edema, and RUQ pain (rule out HELLP syndrome).

Diagnosis:
- Measure blood pressure, urinalysis, urine dipstick, urine microalbumin, and 24-hour urine protein test.
- Need to rule out HELLP syndrome: CBC (anemia/platelets) and LFTs.

Treatment:
- *First step* is to stabilize blood pressure with IV labetalol and/or hydralazine (keep <160/100 mmHg).
- *Next step* is seizure prophylaxis: continuous magnesium sulfate drip.
- Deliver baby after the mother has been stabilized.
- Continue seizure prophylaxis 24 hours postpartum.

<u>Side effects</u> of magnesium sulfate: loss of DTRs and respiratory paralysis.

Eclampsia
Medical emergency

<u>New</u>-onset of grand-mal seizures in women with preeclampsia. Usually last for about a minute.

Hx/PE: Headache, visual changes, RUQ pain, edema, and seizure.

Diagnosis:

- ABCs and stabilization first, then order laboratory tests.
- CBC (platelets/anemia), electrolytes, urinalysis, and LFTs.

Treatment:

- *First steps* are ABCs, oxygen supplementation, IV access, IV fluids, cardiac monitoring, and respiratory monitoring.
- Control blood pressure: IV labetalol and/or hydralazine.
- Magnesium sulfate, 6 g loaded over 15 minutes (less sedative than diazepam and increases cerebral blood flow).
- IV diazepam if seizure recurs.
- Initiate delivery when patient is stable and convulsions are controlled.
- Continue magnesium sulfate for 24 hours after delivery.

Note:

- ✓ Magnesium sulfate toxicity can be reversed with IV calcium gluconate.
- ✓ Deliver when mother is stable and seizures have stopped.

HELLP syndrome

A variant of preeclampsia with poor prognosis that can be life threatening. Patients present with hemolytic anemia, elevated liver enzyme levels, and low platelet count.

Risks factors: age <20 years or >35 years. The only real cure for preeclampsia and eclampsia is delivery.

Complications: aspiration pneumonia, cerebral hemorrhage, hypoxic encephalopathy, prematurity, fetal distress, and seizures.

Hx/PE: RUQ or epigastric abdominal pain, edema, headache, visual changes, elevated blood pressure, seizure, nausea, and vomiting.

Diagnosis:

- CBC (hematocrit [low] and platelets [low]), elevated blood pressure, urinalysis, and liver function test (liver enzymes [high]).

- Hemolysis: measure LDH level, bilirubin level, and serial CBCs.

Treatment:

- The only effective treatment is delivery.
- Anemic patient may require blood transfusion.
- Hypertension is treated with IV labetalol.
- Seizures are treated with bolus plus IV magnesium sulfate.
- If platelets <100,000/mm³, start IV corticosteroids and infuse platelets if <20,000/mm³.
- DIC is treated with FFP.
- If >34 weeks, the baby should be delivered when patient is stabilized and should be given seizure prophylaxis (IV magnesium sulfate).
- If <34 weeks, need to consider immediate expectant management despite fetal status.

Ectopic pregnancy

Ectopic pregnancy

Most common location of ectopic pregnancy is the ampulla. However, ectopic pregnancy can occur in many places. Usually apparent about 6–8 weeks after LMP. If a young patient shows classic symptoms, consider ectopic until proven otherwise.

Risk factors: PID, endometriosis, previous ectopic pregnancies, pelvic surgery, and DES.

Hx/PE: Triad: amenorrhea, vaginal spotting, and lower abdominal pain. Pain felt can be similar to other medical emergencies such as ovarian torsion and appendicitis.

Diagnosis:

- *First test* for stable patients is serial hCG level testing, with observation of appropriate doubling in 48 hour.

- Transvaginal ultrasonography (*more specific*) or transabdominal ultrasonography (*less specific*). These tests help detect pregnancy outside of the uterus.
- Cross matching and Rh factor testing for mother.

Note: intrauterine pregnancies might not be seen by ultrasound until hCG levels reach at least 1,500 IU/L.

Treatment:
- If <u>small</u> (<3.5 cm) and unruptured, give MTX.
- If <u>larger</u> (>3.5 cm), consider **salpingectomy** (if ruptured) or **salpingostomy** (if not ruptured). These procedures cause risk of future ectopic pregnancies.
- Tubal rupture (obstetric emergency), will need laparoscopy/ salpingectomy (removal of fallopian tube).
- Give RhoGam to Rh-negative mothers.

Note: suspect ruptured ectopic pregnancy with presentation of peritoneal irritation, abdominal guarding, or rigidity.

Placental complications

Placental abruption

Premature separation of the placenta from the uterus.

<u>Risk factors</u>: hypertension, infection, trauma, smoking, cocaine, and previous abruptions. If secondary to trauma, there is a 20% probability of developing DIC.

Hx/PE: Lower abdominal pain, dark vaginal bleeding, uterine hypertonicity, and fetal distress.

Diagnosis:
- Clinical diagnosis.
- CBC, electrolytes, Rh factor, type and screen, PTT, PT/INR, and platelet count.
- Fetal heart monitoring, transabdominal ultrasonography (*less stressful*) or transvaginal ultrasonography (*more stressful*).

Treatment:

- In situations of a term fetus consider delivery.

- If mother and fetus are stable and fetus is preterm can consider monitoring in the hospital (IV access, IV fluids, oxygen, fetal monitoring, bed rest, and if needed RhoGam).

- Might need to consider steroids (lung maturity) and GBS prophylaxis.

- Delivery will depend on stability and extent of the placental abruption. Vaginal delivery is the preferred method if mother and fetus are stable.

- Order PRBC on stand-by.

Complications: hemorrhagic shock or DIC (most common complication). If coagulopathy develops, treat with FFP and platelet transfusion.

Placenta previa

Abnormally low placental implantation with classic presentation of "painless bright red vaginal bleeding." A common presentation is bleeding after sexual intercourse; usually no fetal distress on monitoring.

Types:

➤ Total placenta previa (covers os).

➤ Marginal placenta previa (margin of os).

➤ Low placenta previa (near proximity of os).

Risk factors: prior C-sections, prior placenta previa, advanced age, PID, smoking, and multiple gestations.

Diagnosis:

- Transabdominal ultrasonography should be performed *first* followed by transvaginal ultrasonography to determine precise location.

- Digital examination should never be performed prior to abdominal ultrasonography. In fact, they are rarely done with placenta previa.

Note: intravaginal ultrasonography is more accurate than a transabdominal ultrasonography.

Treatment:

- If needed, stabilize the patient and consider administration of tocolytics, betamethasone (fetal lung maturity), and GBS prophylaxis. However, GBS prophylaxis is more commonly indicated for vaginal deliveries.
- Delivery by C-section (absolute indication) unless placenta is >2 cm away from the internal os.
- Deliver if lung maturity is achieved, fetus >36 weeks, or fetal/maternal distress.

<u>Complications</u>: **placenta accreta** (placenta attached to the myometrium), **vasa previa** (obstruction of the fetal blood vessels), PROM, and preterm delivery.

Note: vasa previa can be seen on ultrasonography (vessels crossing over the internal cervical os).

Gestational trophoblastic disease

Can present as a <u>benign</u> (**hydatidiform moles**) or <u>malignant</u> (**choriocarcinoma**) condition.

- ➤ **Complete mole**: two-sperm fertilization of empty egg (46 XX). No fetal tissue.
- ➤ **Incomplete mole** or **partial mole**: ovum is fertilized by two sperms (69 XXY). Has fetal tissue.

Hx/PE: First trimester uterine bleeding (most common), hyperemesis gravidarum, uterine size greater than normal for gestation age. Extreme ages: >40 or <20 years. Diet deficiency of folic acid or β-carotene.

Diagnosis:

- No FHR on Doppler.
- Increase in β-hCG level (usually >100,000 U/mL).
- Pelvic ultrasonography ("**snowstorm**" appearance; no gestational sac or fetus present).

- Pelvic examination ("**grapelike molar cluster**" in the vagina).
- D&C (mass appears like a "**cluster of grapes**").

Treatment:

- Evacuate uterus (D&C).
- Monitor weekly β-hCG levels (to rule out **choriocarcinoma**). If the level shows a decrease, repeat hCG test every month for the next year.
- If hCG levels plateaus over 3 weeks or increase over 2 weeks, give single-dose of MTX. These laboratory findings are more along the lines of choriocarcinoma.
- The patient cannot get pregnant for a year because elevation in hCG levels can be caused by either pregnancy or choriocarcinoma.
- Place the patient on OCPs for a year and evaluate hCG levels during this time frame.

Intrauterine growth restriction (IUGR)

EFW <10 percentile for gestational age or <2.5 kg.

Risk factors: hypertension (most common), substance abuse, chromosomal abnormalities, placenta previa, multiple gestations, and medication use.

➤ Symmetric IUGR: caused by *intrinsic factors* (infection or genetic abnormalities).

➤ Asymmetric IUGR: caused by *extrinsic factors* (malnutrition, alcohol, or tobacco).

Diagnosis:

- *First step* is physical examination with a fundal height measurement (suspect if fundal height is >3 cm smaller than the gestational age).
- *Next step* is pelvic ultrasonography to confirm fetal dates and monitor fetal heart rate.
  - If gestational age is >13 weeks, one of the most accurate measurements is abdominal circumference.

- Monitor, as needed with NST, CST, ultrasonography, BPP, and umbilical artery Doppler velocimetry.

Treatment:
- Explore etiology and administer betamethasone (if needed) to accelerate fetal lung maturity.
- If near term consider prompt vaginal delivery, if no contraindications.

Note: always keep in mind the following during the delivery:

✓ Premature, administer betamethasone (2 dosages over 24 hours).

✓ Rh-negative mother, administer RhoGam.

✓ GBS prophylaxis (amoxicillin or penicillin at least 4 hours before delivery).

Polyhydramnios

AFI >20cm on ultrasonography (measure all 4 quadrants and add volumes).

<u>Risk factors</u>: fetal chromosomal abnormalities, diabetic mother, multiple gestation, duodenal atresia, TE-fistula, and anencephaly.

Diagnosis:
- Physical examination: fundal height higher than expected.
- Ultrasound: AFI >20 cm.
- Rule out GI abnormalities, diabetes, and chromosomal abnormalities.

Treatment: Etiology specific.

<u>Complications</u>: **umbilical cord prolapse** (umbilical cord comes out of the uterus causing cord compression), preterm delivery, and fetal malpresentation.

Oligohydramnios

AFI <5 cm on ultrasonography (measure all 4 quadrants and add volumes). Common with IUGR and fetal distress.

Risk factors: inaccurate gestational dating, urinary tract abnormalities, renal agenesis, and renal obstructions.

Diagnosis:

- Ultrasonography: AFI <5 cm.
- Rule out inaccurate gestational dates and renal problems.
- If asymptomatic, check biweekly fetal BPP.

Treatment: Etiology specific.

Complications: IUGR, clubfoot, muscular skeletal abnormalities, and umbilical cord compression.

Multiple gestations

➢ Monozygotic (rare): identical twins.

➢ Dizygotic (65%) fraternal twins.

Hx/PE: Rapid uterine growth with excessive maternal weight gain.

Diagnosis:

- Ultrasonography (confirmatory) and fetal heart monitoring.
- Elevated hCG, MS-AFP, and HPL level tests.

Treatment: Management by a high-risk specialist is recommended.

Note: maternal complications with multiple gestations are preeclampsia, preterm birth, placental abruption, and IUGR.

Fetal macrosomia

Fetal weight >90% or birth weight of 4.0–4.5 kg. Newborns are at risk of shoulder dystocia and Erb-Duchenne palsy (upper brachial plexus damage).

Material risks: diabetes (most common cause), maternal obesity, and male fetus.

Diagnosis: Weighing newborn at birth or estimating in utero.

Treatment: Cesarean delivery if weight >4.5 kg (if diabetic) or >5.0 kg (if not diabetic) or elective delivery at 38–40 weeks.

Note: babies born to diabetic mothers have a risk of developing hypoglycemia.

Small gestational age
Symmetric decrease in weight, height, and head circumference.

Hx/PE: Hypothermia, hypoglycemia, hypocalcemia, and hypoxia.

Hydrocephalus
Increased intracranial cerebral spinal fluid (CSF) in the ventricles, resulting in increased pressure in the skull. There are two types of hydrocephalus: **communicating hydrocephalus** and **non-communicating hydrocephalus**.

Hx/PE: Nausea, vomiting, and gaze palsy (which are suggestive of increased intracranial pressure).

Treatment: Ventriculoperitoneal shunting or VP-shunting (there are many types of shunts, but this one is commonly used).

Note: patients with VP-shunts are at risk of infection with *S. epididymis* or *S. pseudomonas*. In case of shunt obstruction, the best step is shunt replacement.

Infections during pregnancy

Urinary tract infections during pregnancy

Can increase risk of pyelonephritis, preterm delivery, and low birth weight.

Diagnosis: Urinalysis (*best initial test*) and urine culture (*most accurate test*). If diagnosed, the patient needs to be screened every month even after treatment.

Note: Do not perform abdominal CT scan and IV pyelogram (unless necessary) to avoid increased exposure of the fetus to radiation.

Treatment:

- *First* UTI during pregnancy: treat for 7 days with antibiotics (nitrofurantoin or cephalexin) and a follow-up urine culture should be performed in 10 days.
- *Second* UTI during pregnancy: re-treat for 7 days with the same antibiotics and place on prophylactic antibiotics with nitrofurantoin daily.
- If patient develops pyelonephritis: hospitalize with IV antibiotics (ceftriaxone); once better (afebrile), discharge home on oral antibiotics (14 days).

Prevention: drink 6-8 glasses of water a day, vitamin C (250-500 mg/day), urinate before and after intercourse, and urinate as soon as possible with urgency.

Note: do not use SMP-TMX (decrease folic acid) or fluoroquinolones (damage cartilage).

Bacterial vaginosis in pregnancy

Diagnosis: Physical examination "fishy odor" and microscopic examination [wet mount] clue cells.

Treatment: Treat with oral metronidazole or clindamycin for 7 days.

Note:

- Lesbian sexual partners have an increased risk of bacterial vaginosis.
- Can treat infection with *Trichomonas vaginalis in pregnancy* also with metronidazole (one dose only).
- A breastfeeding mother should discontinue breastfeeding for 24-hours while on metronidazole and provide the baby with nutrition supplementation.

Chorioamnionitis

Commonly caused by <u>ascending</u> vaginal flora bacteria such as GBS and *E. coli*. Can also be caused by prolonged labor and increased vaginal examinations during the final months of pregnancy.

<u>Risk factors</u>: amniocentesis and vaginal procedures.

Hx/PE: Maternal fever, foul smelling amniotic fluid, and uterine tenderness; caused by a number of infections.

Diagnosis: Clinical diagnosis (fever, leukocytosis, and uterine tenderness).

Treatment:

- Treat as soon as possible, can lead to maternal or neonatal infection.
- Administer antibiotics:
  - <u>Standard treatment:</u> ampicillin plus gentamycin.
  - <u>C-section delivery</u>: use ampicillin plus gentamycin and clindamycin.

Endometritis

Referred to as inflammation of the endometrium (inter lining of uterus). Postpartum endometritis is usually caused by polymicrobial infection.

<u>Risk factors:</u> the highest risk factor for development of endometritis is C-section. Can also be caused by PROM, prolonged labor, and multiple vaginal examinations.

Hx/PE: Fever, uterine tenderness, and malodorous lochia.

Diagnosis:

- Fever, leukocytosis, uterine tenderness, and malodorous lochia.
- Need to rule out sepsis with blood cultures.
- After delivery, consider pelvic CT scan (to check for abscesses).

Treatment:

- **Endometritis**: hospitalize and start IV antibiotics: clindamycin and gentamicin (gold standard), until afebrile for 48 hours <u>or</u> 24 hours for **chorioamnionitis**.
- Add ampicillin for complicated cases.
- Use anticoagulation with heparin for 7 to 10 days (for septic pelvic thrombophlebitis).

Note: postpartum fever that is <u>not</u> responsive to antibiotics, consider **septic pelvic thrombophlebitis** leading to septic embolization (abdominal pain and "**picket-fence**" fevers with a body temperature as high as 41°C).

Mastitis

A type of cellulitis caused by nipple trauma or *S. aureus* infection from the infant's pharynx. Usually begins 2–4 weeks postpartum.

Hx/PE: Usually unilateral, erythema, edema, warmth, and possible purulent nipple drainage.

Diagnosis: Clinical diagnosis; can conduct a breast milk culture (increased WBC).

Note: if suspected, need to rule out breast cancer with mastitis.

Treatment:

- Continued breastfeeding helps remove infected material <u>or</u> a breast pump (not as effective as breastfeeding) can be used.
- PO antibiotics: treat with penicillin antibiotics (**dicloxacillin**) or azithromycin, if allergic to penicillin.
- If an abscess develops (confirm with ultrasound) and then incision and drainage should be performed.

Note: dicloxacillin is different from doxycycline (which is contraindicated).

Herpes during pregnancy

➤ If risk of active herpes close to the time of birth, give the patient prophylactic acyclovir starting at 36 weeks.

➤ Mother with active genital lesions during labor, C-section is indicated.

Chlamydia during pregnancy

Chlamydia is a common STD caused by bacterium Chlamydia trachomatis.

Diagnosis:

- Papanicolaou test with vaginal culture and PCR testing (*gold standard*).
- Urine rapid test with PCR (*rapid means*). Can purchase these over the counter.

Treatment: Oral azithromycin 1g single dose or oral erythromycin 500 mg q4/d for 7 days. Need to give IM ceftriaxone to cover gonorrhea.

Note: do not use tetracycline's or fluoroquinolones during pregnancy.

Hepatitis B positive mother

➤ If the mother is <u>immune</u> to hepatitis B, only the recommended dose of hepatitis B vaccination needs to be given to the neonates.

➤ If the mother is positive and <u>non-immune</u> to hepatitis B, the newborn will need <u>both</u> hepatitis B vaccination and hepatitis B immune globulin within 12 hours.

➤ Keep in mind that neonates have a higher risk of developing chronic hepatitis (about 80%) as opposed to acquiring hepatitis as an adult.

➤ Breastfeeding is <u>not</u> contraindicated for children with mothers with hepatitis B. However, neonates will need to receive the vaccination first.

- A mother with hepatitis B can deliver the neonate vaginally and <u>not</u> an indication for cesarean section.
- Avoid invasive procedures (e.g., CVS).

Tuberculosis in pregnancy

- Positive pregnant mothers can be treated with triple therapy for 6 months: INH, rifampin, ethambutol, and B6
- In case of positive PPD and negative chest radiography, use INH and B6 for 9 months.
- <u>Cannot</u> use pyrazinamide or streptomycin, since these medications are teratogenic.
- If infant develops TB meningitis, treatment is required for 12 months.
- Contraindicated to breastfeed neonate with active TB.

Prophylaxis during pregnancy

Rh isoimmunization

Caused by fetal RBCs leaking into the maternal circulation and the transfer of maternal anti-Rh IgG antibodies to the placenta, leading to hemolysis of fetal Rh (erythroblastosis fetalis). Can cause fetal hypoxia and death.

Risk factors: Rh-negative status or previous deliveries without RhoGAM.

Diagnosis: Rh-negative mother can be monitored by serial ultrasonography and amniocentesis can be performed for evidence of fetal hemolysis.

Treatment:

- A 300-mcg prophylactic dose of RhoGAM should be administered at the 28th week of gestation and again at delivery.

- In severe cases, initiate preterm delivery when the lungs have matured.
- **Intrauterine blood transfusion** can be performed to correct low fetal hematocrit.

Prevention:

- Give Rh-negative mother RhoGAM at 28 weeks and within 72 hours of delivery.
- Give RhoGAM to Rh-negative mothers in the following cases: abortion, ectopic pregnancy, CVS, amniocentesis, vaginal bleeding, placenta previa, or placental abruption.
- Rh isoimmunization causes more severe complications than ABO incompatibility.

Complications: hydrops fetalis (fetal hemoglobin drops to <7 g/dL).

Group B streptococcus (GBS)

A type of bacteria found in the vagina, bladder, or rectum of pregnant women. This bacterium can cause infection postpartum in neonates such as meningitis and sepsis. More commonly transmitted via vaginal delivery, as compared to C-section.

Diagnosis: Can screen women at 37 weeks for GBS; if results are not available, give prophylaxis at birth.

Treatment:

- Chemoprophylaxis with intrapartum IV penicillin G or ampicillin is considered adequate if given 4 hours prior to delivery.
- If not adequately treated, observe for at least 48 hours.
- No need for GBS prophylaxis, if planned C-section without rupture of membrane (despite culture results).

Note: If allergic to penicillin, use clindamycin.

Fetal malpresentation

Breech

Presentation of the fetus in a position other than the vertex position with chin to chest and occiput anterior.

Breech risk factors: premature birth, prior breech, polyhydramnios, oligohydramnios, placenta previa, and multiple gestations.

Diagnosis:

- **Frank breech**: (*most common*) thighs flexed and knees extended.
- **Complete breech**: thighs flexed and knees flexed.
- **Footing breech**: one or both legs are below the buttocks.
- **Compound presentation**: hand near the head or many other possibilities. Can still have vaginal delivery in most cases.

Treatment:

- >85% of breech presentations will become vertex by 36 weeks.
- **External cephalic version**: applying direct pressure on the abdomen can help change the fetal position (to the cephalic position). Usually, done at about 37 weeks.

  Contraindications for external cephalic version:
  - Once labor has started.
  - Abnormal fetal heart tracing.
  - Low amniotic fluid level.
- Emergency C-section or elective C-section (if low risk of morbidity).

  Complications: cord compression and placental abruption.

Twin delivery presentations

➤ Babies either both in vertex/vertex position, vertex/transverse position, or vertex/breech position.

- If baby <u>A</u> is in the vertex position, mother can decide mode of delivery (vaginal or C-section).
- If both in non-vertex positions, C-section delivery is generally recommended.
- If first twin is delivered and labor is halted then, give oxytocin if no contraindications.
- Usually delivered by a twin specialist.

Cesarean section

Indications for cesarean section

- <u>Maternal factors</u>: cephalopelvic disproportion (most common), HIV infection (>1,000 viral load), prior *vertical* C-section (*transverse* is a relative indication), active vaginal herpes, cervical carcinoma, total placenta previa (unless placenta >2 cm from internal os), failed vaginal delivery, and post-term pregnancy (relative).
- <u>Fetal factors</u>: malpresentation (shoulder presentation, breech, posterior chin, or transverse), fetal distress, cord compression, and erythroblastosis fetalis. Fetal scalp pH <7.2 requires delivery.

Note: transverse C-sections is not an absolute contraindication but carries increased risk of hemorrhage and rupture.

Treatment: Give **sodium citrate** before cesarean delivery to decrease gastric acidity and prevent aspiration syndrome.

Note: patients with previous caesarean section, attempting vaginal delivery and presenting with rapid deterioration, decreased strength of contractions, and hemodynamic instability, rule out **intra-abdominal hemorrhage** caused by uterine rupture (**medical emergency**). Common among patients with previous C-section.

Postpartum complications

Postpartum hemorrhage

Acceptable blood loss during delivery is <500 mL (vaginal) or <1000 mL (C-section). Can occur before, during, or after delivery. If greater than these values, the patient is at risk of Sheehan's syndrome.

Risk factors: **Sheehan's syndrome** (pituitary ischemia): leads to damage of the pituitary and failure to lactate (prolactin).

Uterine atony: most common cause of postpartum hemorrhage (90%); also caused by macrosomia, polyhydramnios, or multiple gestations.

Diagnosis:

- *Uterine atony*: soft, enlarged, boggy uterus accompanied by postpartum hemorrhage of >500 ml.

- *Sheehan's syndrome*: measure TSH, prolactin levels, and pituitary MRI (rule out tumors).

Treatment:

- Uterine atony:

    - *First line*: uterine massage.

    - *Second line*: oxytocin.

    - *Third line*: **methergine** (if not hypertensive/preeclampsia); need to check blood pressure. Can also use prostaglandin (PGF2α), which is contraindicated in asthmatics.

    - If unsuccessful, uterine artery ligation can be performed.

- Sheehan's syndrome: lifelong hormone replacement with deficient hormones.

Genital tract trauma

Risk factors: forceps, vacuum, large infant, first child, and inadequate episiotomy repair.

Diagnosis: Manual or visual inspection (look for lacerations >2 cm).

Treatment: If >2 cm or uncontrolled bleeding, perform surgical repair.

Note: vacuum-assisted or forceps-assisted delivery is not to be performed at a station higher than +2 (including all negative numbers [-3, -2, -1]) and mother needs to be fully dilated (second stage of labor). Vacuum assistance cannot be given in case of face presentation.

Episiotomy

➤ **Median episiotomy** (midline): risk of extension to the anal sphincter (3rd degree and 4th degree).

➤ **Mediolateral episiotomy**: risk of increased bleeding.

Retained placental tissue

Considered retained if the placental tissue has not detached from the uterus within 30 minutes of stage 3 labor. This can lead to uterine hemorrhage and infection.

Diagnosis: Manual or visual inspection <u>plus</u> ultrasonography may be used to inspect the uterus.

Treatment: Manual removal and/or curettage with genital suctioning.

Sheehan's syndrome

Postpartum pituitary ischemia/necrosis caused by obstetric hemorrhage or shock, which presents with failure to lactate because of decreased prolactin release.

Hx/PE: May present with other pituitary symptoms such as hypothyroidism, adrenal insufficiency, diabetes insipidus (DI), amenorrhea, and inability to lactate.

Diagnosis: Hormonal testing (TSH and prolactin levels), and head MRI (pituitary and hypothalamus) to rule out tumors or other pathologies.

Treatment:

- Replacement of all deficient hormones.
- Cortisol can be helpful in recovering some hormones.

ABO blood group incompatibility

Risk when mother is type O+ with type A or B infant (not the other way around). Common symptoms are <u>mild</u> hemolysis and jaundice.

Mitral stenosis and pregnancy

Can be an indication for forceps assisted delivery (at stage 2 of labor) to help decrease maternal valsalva efforts and maternal tachycardia.

Endocarditis prophylaxis

Needed during labor for vaginal delivery or C-section, if there is a history of endocarditis or prosthetic heart valve.

Postpartum lochia

Normal process of vaginal fluid changing from bright red blood, to pinkish-brown, to yellow-white blood. Lochia can last up to 6 weeks after childbirth and is completely normal.

Multiparous

Is defined as giving birth >2 times and can cause pelvic dysfunction leading to urinary and/or fecal incontinence or constipation.

DVT medications during pregnancy

➤ Discontinue warfarin and start SQ heparin injections daily.

➤ Warfarin is contraindicated during pregnancy (category X medication).

➤ Warfarin is not contraindicated during breastfeeding.

Postpartum thyroiditis

➤ Autoimmune in nature and does <u>not</u> cause thyroid tenderness or enlargement.

➤ Resolves by 1-week to 1-year postpartum and can progress to permanent hypothyroidism.

➤ Drug of choice for hypothyroidism is levothyroxine.

➤ Drug of choice for hyperthyroidism are β-blockers and PTU (first trimester) and methimazole (second and third trimester).

Note: never use radioactive iodine during pregnancy.

Birth control postpartum

➤ Lactating mothers should be given progestin only OCPs (Depo-Provera or Implanon). This will not decrease milk production and is an effective contraceptive.

➤ IUDs should be deferred for at least 6 weeks postpartum.

➤ If given combination OCPs (estrogen containing) lactation will decrease, as estrogen inhibits prolactin.

➤ Breastfeeding alone can be successful in the first 6 months, especially if baby is exclusively breastfeeding. After 6 months when the baby is being supplemented with solids, this form of birth control becomes less effective.

Precautions during pregnancy

➤ All pregnant drivers should wear seatbelts with both lap and shoulder straps.

➤ Scuba diving is <u>not</u> recommended during pregnancy.

➤ Patients on levothyroxine, the dosage often needs to be increased.

➤ Patients on insulin, the dosage often needs to be increased.

➤ Always educate patients on drugs, smoking, and alcohol usage.

➤ Need to review all medications given during pregnancy.

Breastfeeding

Lactation and breastfeeding

➤ During pregnancy, increased estrogen and progesterone causes <u>inhibition</u> of prolactin.

➤ After delivery, estrogen and progesterone drop and suckling leads to increase in prolactin (milk let down) and oxytocin (milk ejection).

➤ Benefits of breastfeeding are decreased likelihood of newborn allergies, URI, and GI infections. Helps with bonding between mother and child, and helps with maternal weight loss.

➤ Breast milk contains IgA.

<u>Contraindications and precautions during breastfeeding</u>:

- Breastfeeding is contraindicated for mothers with HIV, active or untreated tuberculosis, and active herpes virus on the breast. Also in patients taking tetracycline or chloramphenicol.

- Diagnosis of galactosemia is a contraindication for breastfeeding.

- Current studies show that warfarin is <u>not</u> contraindicated during breastfeeding (but is contraindicated during pregnancy).

- Anti-epileptic medications are <u>not</u> contraindicated during breastfeeding.

- Lactating women who receive metronidazole should discontinue breastfeeding for at least 24 hours and continue thereafter.

Note: there is <u>no</u> risk factor of breastfeeding for mothers with HCV.

Colostrum (early breast milk): contains IgA (passive immunity), high in fat, and proteins.

Post-partum psychology

Post-partum blues

Start immediately after birth and last about 2 weeks; normal in about 1/3rd of all mothers postpartum. Patient presents with sadness, mild fatigue, and tearfulness. Mother does care for her baby.

Treatment: Supportive and usually self-limiting.

Postpartum depression

Within 1–3 months postpartum, major depression lasting longer than 7 days. Patient may want to hurt baby.

Hx/PE: Depressed mood, weight changes, and sleep disturbances, and negative feelings towards the baby in some cases.

Treatment:

- Psychotherapy and anti-depressant medications (SSRIs).
- Severe depression: use ECT (safe during pregnancy and treatment of choice in suicidal patients).

Postpartum psychosis

Within 2–3 weeks postpartum; auditory or visual hallucination often with infanticide ideations and possible suicidal thoughts.

Treatment:

- Risperidone, lithium, and possible anti-depressants.
- If breastfeeding, then ECT is optimal.

Gynecology

Puberty

Introduction

<u>Stages</u>:

➤ <u>Females</u>: most females reach puberty between the ages of 8 and 14 years, with 11 years being the average age for puberty onset. Puberty in females is usually marked by thelarche (breast development) which is the first sign of puberty, followed by adrenarche (axillary hair), and increase in weight and height. Menarche (start of menses) occurs between the age of 10 and 13 years.

➤ <u>Males</u>: most males reach puberty between the age of 9 and 14 years, with 12 years being the average age for puberty onset. Puberty in males is usually marked by testicular enlargement followed by adrenarche and increase in weight and height.

Precocious puberty: defined as females and males reaching puberty before the ages of 8 and 9 years, respectively.

Delayed puberty: females with **no** breast development by the age of 13 years and males with **no** testicular growth by the age of 14 years.

Note: pubertal gynecomastia is seen in about 50% of the males and is considered normal; no further work-up is needed. This is caused by elevated estrogen levels during this time.

- Evaluation for delayed puberty, if no thelarche by 13 years or no menarche by 15 years.
- Work-up is complicated and includes measuring gonadotropins (FSH and LH), hCG, estradiol, testosterone, GnRH, TSH, sonography, head MRI, karyotype, and bone age.

Treatment:

- Treatment depends on pathology.
- Might require treatment with appropriate hormone replacement: Males (testosterone) and females (estrogen and progesterone). Consider growth hormone.

Menstruation

➤ **Follicular phase** (proliferative phase) {days 1–13}: increase in FSH → growth of follicle → increase in estrogen.

➤ **Ovulation phase** {day 14}: LH and FSH spike rupture of follicle and release of mature ovum.

➤ **Luteal phase** (secretory phase) {days 15–28}: corpus luteum cannot survive without further LH stimulation.

- Corpus luteum produces estrogen and progesterone, which peak at day 21.
- Endometrial lining is thickened and releases thick secretions.
- If the corpus luteum does not undergo implantation, it develops into corpus albicans (scar tissue).

Note: Mid-cycle progesterone is a great way to check for ovulation.

Mittelschmerz

Pelvic pain occurs during **ovulation** (mid-cycle) when the follicle ruptures. The pathology is not completely understood but appears to be caused by follicular swelling of the ovarian wall. The pain can appear similar to appendicitis, menstrual cramps, or ovarian pathology.

Hx/PE: _Unilateral_ pelvic pain (ovary rupture) mid-cycle.

Diagnosis: Pelvic examination (to rule out pathology), pelvic ultrasonography, and hCG level.

Treatment: NSAIDs (pain and inflammation) or OCPs (inhibit ovulation).

Note:

    ✓ **Menstrual** **cramps** are mid-pelvic pain that start before the period starts.

    ✓ Mittelschmerz is unilateral pain, arising from the ovary that is ovulating.

Menstrual cramps

Caused by increased prostaglandin release (PGE-2), which causes uterine smooth muscle contractions.

<u>Types:</u>

    ➤ **Primary** dysmenorrhea: no underlying pathology.

    ➤ **Secondary** dysmenorrhea: underlying pathology.

Hx/PE: <u>Mid</u>-pelvic pain (uterus contracting), back pain, nausea, vomiting that occurs a few days before the period starts.

Diagnosis: Will need work-up with Pap smear, abdominal ultrasonography, and serum hCG.

Treatment:

- First line treatment NSAIDs and hot compresses.
- Can also consider OCPs, to control hormonal levels.

Premenstrual dysphoric disorder (PMDD)

PMDD is a **severe** disease that involves physical and emotional symptoms that can effect personal relationships and disrupt daily functioning. Symptoms start 1-2 weeks before menstruation and subside with menstruation. **Premenstrual syndrome (PMS)** is the same as PMDD except a milder form. They increase lifetime risk of psychiatric disorder such as depression or anxiety.

Diagnosis:

- Clinical diagnosis; no further work-up is needed.
- Must have **emotional** symptoms during the luteal phase of menstruation.

Treatment: SSRIs (first line), vitamin B6, OCPs, and psychotherapy.

Note: If one type of SSRI is not effective, then switch to another SSRI.

Amenorrhea

Primary amenorrhea

Lack of spontaneous uterine bleeding by the age of 16 years, which can manifest with or without secondary development.

a. **Without** secondary development (no estrogen present):

- ➤ **Constitutional growth delay**: most common type of primary amenorrhea, caused by delayed puberty.
- ➤ **Kallmann syndrome**: amenorrhea caused by hypogonadotropic hypogonadism (absence of GnRH). Can include anosmia, amenorrhea, color blindness, and facial deformities.

b. **With** secondary characteristics (presence of estrogen production): look for other genetic or anatomic problems.

- ➤ **Mullerian agenesis**: absence of Mullerian ducts, causing absence of upper 1/3rd of the vagina, uterus, and ovarian tubes. The lower 2/3rd of the vagina and ovaries are present (normal estrogen and testosterone levels).
- ➤ **Complete androgen insensitivity**: aromatization of testosterone to estrogen. Normal female phenotype (enlarged hips, small breasts, and female fat tissue distribution) with male genotype (46XY). Usually have sparse genital hair, no uterus, and normal male testosterone levels. Poses increased risk of testicular tumors and undescended testes should be removed.

Diagnosis:

- hCG level (first step in amenorrhea).
- Measure bone age: (radiography):
  - In those aged <12 years and showing normal growth velocity, it is most likely constitutional growth delay.
  - In those aged >12 years and with no signs of puberty, check GnRH, LH, FSH, progesterone, estrogen, and testosterone.
- Measure GnRH, LH, FSH, estrogen, progesterone, and testosterone:
  - Low levels of GnRH, LH, and FSH (*hypogonadotropic hypogonadism)* could be secondary to constitutional growth delay, Kallmann syndrome, hypothalamic, or pituitary problem.
  - High levels of GnRH, LH, FSH, and low estrogen/progesterone (*hypergonadotropic hypogonadism*) indicate ovarian failure to produce estrogen.
  - High levels of GnRH, LH, FSH, and high testosterone or estrogen, are suggestive of PCOS or defective estrogen receptors.
  - Normal levels of GnRH, LH, FSH, and estrogen are suggestive of obstructive problems and imperforated hymen.

If you suspect:

- **Turner syndrome**: obtain karyotype (XO) and estrogen levels.
- **Androgen insensitivity syndrome**: obtain karyotype (XY) and testosterone levels.
- **Imperforated hymen**: conduct vaginal examination.
- **Asherman syndrome**: conduct pelvic ultrasonography, laparoscopy, and hysteroscopy (gold standard).
- **CNS pathology**: perform head MRI with pituitary protocol.
- **PCOS**: conduct pelvic ultrasonography and check GnRH, FSH, and LH levels.

Treatment:

- **Constitutional growth delay**, observation is sufficient (follow-up in 3 months).

- **Turner syndrome**, administer estrogen plus progesterone therapy and growth hormone.
- **Imperforated hymen**, administer first line (OCPs and NSAIDs) and second line intervention (**hymenotomy**).
- **Asherman syndrome**, adhesion dissection will be required.
- **Mullerian agenesis**, consideration of surgical elongation of vagina.

Secondary amenorrhea

Absence of menstrual period for 3–6 cycles in women who previously had normal or irregular periods.

➤ Previously **regular** menses, the patient can be diagnosed with secondary amenorrhea after 3 months.

➤ Previously **irregular** menses, the patient can be diagnosed with secondary amenorrhea after 6 months.

Types:

➤ Pregnancy (most common cause), menopause, breastfeeding, drug induced, and hypothyroidism.

➤ Central hypogonadism: caused by many factors, including malnutrition, anorexia nervosa, stress, excess exercise, and CNS tumors (prolactinemia).

➤ Imperforate hymen: blood cannot escape because of obstruction of hymen.

➤ Asherman syndrome: amenorrhea caused by intrauterine adhesions. Usually secondary to dilation and curettage (D&C) and uterine infections (pelvic inflammatory disease, PID).

Diagnosis:
- First obtain hCG level.
- If negative hCG results are obtained, measure TSH and prolactin levels.
    - Elevated prolactin level can be attributed to hypothyroidism (order TSH).
    - Elevated prolactin level can also be attributed to pituitary tumor (order pituitary MRI).

- If TSH and prolactin are at normal levels, perform a progesterone withdrawal test (IM or oral progesterone for 5 to 10 days and look for withdrawal menstrual bleeding).

- **Progesterone challenge test**: positive bleeding indicates no progesterone. If there is no bleeding, perform an **estrogen-progesterone challenge test**: positive bleeding indicates decreased estrogen. If low in either case, check LH and FSH. If there is no bleeding after estrogen-progesterone challenge, it is most likely Asherman syndrome.

Treatment:

- Hypothalamic (absence of GnRH): give GnRH analogs.

- Small pituitary tumor (prolactinemia): give cabergoline or bromocriptine.

- Large pituitary tumor and not relieved by medications then consider surgical excision.

- Hypothyroidism: Give levothyroxine.

- Premature ovarian failure: estrogen plus progestin replacement therapy.

Dysfunctional uterine bleeding (DUB)

Caused by abnormal hormone levels; **unopposed** estrogen leads to endometrial proliferation, resulting in a random breakdown of endometrial tissue in an irregular and unpredictable manner. The uterine lining exceeds blood supply and causes sloughing of the tissue.

Diagnosis:

- CBC (rule out anemia), iron levels (rule out iron deficiency), pelvic ultrasonography (rule out pathology), and hCG (rule out pregnancy).

- Order: PT/INR, PTT, bleeding time, and type and screen.

Treatment:

- **If stable**: OCPs (regulates estrogen levels) **or** oral cyclic progestin on days 14–25 of the cycle.

- **If unstable**: ABCs, hospitalize, iron supplementation, IV fluids, IV estrogen 25mg (q4-6 hours) until bleeding stops.

- If treatment fails, consider D&C or hysterectomy.
- Hospitalization is required if hematocrit <10 g/dL despite being hemodynamically stable.

Note: If patient is unstable: evaluate ABCs, fluid status, and start IV estrogen.

Menopause

A normal mid-life change in a female's reproductive life. Described as cessation of menses for a minimum of 12 months. Inability to release eggs from the ovaries, secondary to an abnormal response of the ovaries to hormones (FSH and LH). Average age of onset is 51 years.

Premature menopause is defined as menopause **before** the age of 40 years.

Hx/PE: Increased risk of osteoporosis, cardiovascular disease, increase in LDL, mood change, hot flashes, dyspareunia, loss of libido, insomnia, vaginal dryness, and **vaginal atrophy** (caused by low estrogen levels, which manifest as dyspareunia and vaginal bleeding after intercourse).

Diagnosis:
- Clinical diagnosis (history and physical examination).
- Rule out hCG, TSH, and prolactin.
- Elevated FSH (levels increase first) and LH (levels increase later), and low serum estradiol.
- Irregular uterine bleeding and >45 years require endometrial biopsy to rule out endometrial hyperplasia or endometrial cancer.
- **Inhibin B**: Measures ovarian reserve, which decreases after the age of 35 years.
- **Screening:**
  - Lipid profile:
    - Start screening females at the age of 45 years, if no risk factors.
    - In case of risk factors (hypertension, diabetes, or obesity), start screening earlier.

- Re-screen every 5 years, if there are no risk factors and yearly, if there are high risk factors.
- DEXA scan:
  - Start screening at the age of 65 years, if there are no risk factors.
  - If starting chronic steroids **or** in case of fractures out of proportion with trauma, order DEXA scan earlier.

Treatment:

- **First line**: short duration of hormone replacement therapy (HRT), i.e., combination of estrogen and progestin, which are mainly used to treat hot flashes.
- **Second line**: clonidine is used to treat hot flashes but has no osteoporotic benefits.
- Vaginal estrogen cream can be helpful for vaginal atrophy, itching, and dryness.
  - **Types**:
    - Short term: give estrogen vaginal cream.
    - Long term: give estradiol vaginal rings.
    - Non-HRT: **clonidine** (decreases hot flashes) or **venlafaxine** (decreases hot flashes).
- Post hysterectomy patients do **not** need progestin combination.
- Osteoporosis: daily calcium and vitamin D supplementation, exercise, and bisphosphonates (if severe T-score <2.5).

Side effects of HRT include DVTs (two-fold increase), strokes, heart attacks, endometrial cancer, and breast cancer. Need to taper HRT, **cannot** be abruptly stopped. Always need to review the risks and benefits. Administer HRT for a short duration and at the lowest dose possible.

Contraindications of HRT: high risk of breast cancer, endometrial cancer, history of thromboembolism, chronic liver disease, or hypertriglyceridemia.

Contraceptives

Combination Oral Contraceptives

Mechanism of action: inhibits FSH/LH (suppressing ovulation).

Can improve: acne, dysmenorrhea, regulates menstrual periods, PCOS, menstrual cramps, PMS, and adenomyosis. Decrease risk of ovarian cancer and ectopic pregnancies.

Risk factors: thromboembolism especially in women >35 year of age who smoke. Can cause break through bleeding.

Absolute contraindications: pregnancy, DVT, factor V Leiden, PE, stroke, liver disease (hepatocarcinoma), uncontrolled hypertension, breast cancer, uterine cancer, migraine headache **with** aura, stage 2 hypertension (160/100 mm Hg), and undiagnosed vaginal bleeding.

Note:

✓ Combination OCPs do **not** cause weight gain.

✓ Can cause OCP-induced hypertension.

✓ Anti seizure medications (induce cytochrome P450) decrease efficacy of OCPs.

✓ Rule out pregnancy before prescribing any contraceptive.

Transdermal contraceptive patch

Combined estrogen and progestin dermal patch that needs to be changed weekly.

How to use the patch: place the patch on the skin (leg, buttocks, or arm) each week on the same day and time; remove the old patch and place a new patch for a total of 3 weeks. At the end of the third week, remove the old patch and do not place a new patch until the following week (basically 3 weeks on and 1 week off).

Risks: thromboembolism (especially for women aged over 35 years who smoking), stroke, MI, DVT, hyperlipidemia, liver disease, increased risk of breast cancer, and endometrial cancer.

NuvaRing "the ring"

Low dose progestin and estrogen vaginal ring to be used continuously for 3 weeks and removed for 1 week.

Advantages: helps with acne, dysmenorrhea, pregnancy, vaginal dryness, lighter periods, and regulates periods. Can be used continuously to skip periods (not recommended).

Disadvantages: does not protect against sexually transmitted diseases.

Side effects: spotting is common in the first few months and may experience increased vaginal discharge.

Progestin-only contraceptives

Used postpartum in women who are breastfeeding and do not want to get pregnant, especially when the child is breastfeeding less and supplementation of other foods are introduced. During this time, a mother has an increased risk of becoming pregnant, as breastfeeding is not a reliable contraceptive.

Implanon "the implant"

The progestin-only implant is placed under the skin (subdermal); it lasts up to 3 years. This medication is safe during breastfeeding and the woman can regain fertility soon after removal. Progesterone contraception decreases the risk of endometrial cancer.

Side effects: weight gain, irregular bleeding, and depression.

Depo-Provera (medroxyprogesterone)

IM injected contraceptive that needs to be given every 3 months.

Advantages: safe for breastfeeding mothers and lighter or no periods. No increased risk of DVTs, MI, stroke, or endometrial cancer.

Side effects: delayed fertility after discontinuation, irregular bleeding, weight gain, and decreased bone mineral density.

Note: Depo-Provera has no increased risk of endometrial cancer or DVT because of the lack of an estrogen component.

ParaGard (copper IUD)

A copper-based contraceptive that acts as a spermicide, which is effective for about 10 years. Can obtain fertility soon after removal and is safe during breastfeeding. Intrauterine devices are **more** reliable than OCPs.

Side effects: increased bleeding, perforation of the cervix, increased cramping, discomfort during sexual intercourse, and possible actinomycosis.

Contraindications: unresolved cervical cancer, PID, unexplained vaginal bleeding, Wilson's disease, and pregnancy.

Before usage: always conduct a vaginal culture and pregnancy test before placement.

Male condom

Advantages: covers the penis and protects against most STDs and pregnancy.

Disadvantages: 12% failure rate. Does not protect against herpes or syphilis infections that are on the pubis or other areas that the condom does not cover. For example, a herpes lesion that is not on the penis shaft.

Side effects: possible allergic reaction (latex).

Bilateral vasectomy

Has the **lowest** chance of failure out of all contraceptives other than abstinence.

Other contraceptives: diaphragm, female condom, withdrawal method, spermicide, and fertility awareness method.

Vaginal Infections

Bacterial vaginosis (BV)

Not considered an STD and often caused by changes in vaginal flora (polymicrobic) or vaginal pH. Semen elevates vaginal pH and can exacerbate smell.

Risk factors: pregnancy, semen (controversial), >1 sexual partner, new sexual partner, or female-female partners.

Hx/PE: Increased runny white-greyish vaginal discharge with a fish-like odor.

Diagnosis:

- Pelvic exam and **wet mount**: "Clue cells."
- **Positive whiff test** (before or after placing one drop of 10% KOH on the sample, releases an intense amine odor).
- Vaginal pH >4.5.

Treatment:

- PO or vaginal metronidazole (BID ×7 days) **or** clindamycin. No need to treat sexual partner.
- Pregnancy: Can use **oral** metronidazole or clindamycin. Do not use vaginal antibiotics (less effective).

Note: no studies show that BV causes preterm delivery, unlike trichomoniasis.

Vaginal yeast infection

Risk factors: diabetes, pregnancy, HIV, steroids, antibiotics, OCPs, IUDs, and frequent intercourse.

Hx/PE: Extreme **pruritus** with thick white vaginal discharge, "cottage cheese-like".

Diagnosis:

- Pelvic examination and pap smear.

- pH: 4.0–4.5 and wet mount (hyphae/pseudohyphae with KOH).
- Need to screen for diabetes (fasting glucose).

Treatment:

- Fluconazole orally in a **single** 150 mg dose (best) **or** nystatin intravaginal.
- Miconazole cream intravaginal (7 days) is preferred over oral fluconazole during the first trimester of **pregnancy**.

Sexually transmitted disease

*For more STD details see "Infectious Diseases in Your Pocket"

Trichomoniasis

Is an STD (protozoan family) caused by unprotected sex and increased risk with multiple sexual partners.

Hx/PE: Increased greenish-yellow purulent discharge with a fish-like smell and pruritus.

Diagnosis:

- Pelvic examination: "**Strawberry cervix**" and yellow-green frothy discharge and positive whiff test.
- Wet mount: "**Motile flagellated**" organism.
- Vaginal pH > 4.5.

Treatment:

- Single dose of PO metronidazole (2,000mg).
- Need to treat sexual partner/s (not needed in case of BV).
- A breastfeeding mother should stop breastfeeding for 24 hours after starting treatment with metronidazole. During this time, the mother should use a breast pump to express the milk containing the medication. Need to supplement baby with formula during this time.

Screening: if diagnosed with one STD screen for other STDs.

Note: compare the single dose treatment with trichomoniasis, compared to full week treatment with BV.

Gonorrhea

An STD caused by *N. gonorrhoeae* (gram negative diplococcal) that commonly presents with chlamydia.

Hx/PE: Pelvic pain, dysuria, dyspareunia, and vaginal discharge.

Diagnosis:

- Need to swab patient→ STD panel (culture) with Gram stain (stain shows diplococcal).
- Most sensitive and rapid test is **nucleic acid amplification test** (NAAT). This test can be done with a urine sample.

Treatment:

- Single **IM** dose of ceftriaxone and a single **oral** dose of azithromycin.
- For pregnant patients, switch azithromycin with erythromycin.
- Treat sexual partner/s.

Chlamydia

Most common **bacterial** STD worldwide. The most common **viral** STD is human papilloma virus (HPV). Chlamydia is a gram-negative obligate intracellular microorganism caused by the bacterium *C. trachomatis*.

Hx/PE: Pelvic pain, dysuria, dyspareunia, and vaginal discharge.

Diagnosis: NAATs such as, PCR (very sensitive).

Treatment:

- **Oral** azithromycin (single dose) and **IM** ceftriaxone (single dose).
- PO doxycycline for 7 days is an alternative.
- Treat pregnant patient with oral azithromycin 1g single dose **or** oral erythromycin for 7 days.

Note:

✓ Chlamydia is not diagnostic on Gram stain (mainly detects elevated WBC count).

✓ If mild PID, treat with one dose of IM ceftriaxone and use oral doxycycline for 14 days.

✓ If severe PID, consider IM ceftriaxone and IV use of doxycycline.

Human papilloma virus (HPV)

Most common **viral** STD in the United States. **Condyloma acuminata** is a dermatological manifestation of HPV arising from subtypes 6 and 11. HPV 16, 18, and 31 can cause SCC. Condyloma acuminate is **not** a contraindication for vaginal delivery.

Diagnosis:

- Clinical diagnosis.

- Can use **acetic acid test** to localize lesions **or** biopsy.

- In case of abnormal Pap smear, perform colposcopy and endocervical curettage.

  - **Colposcopy** is useful for viewing the vagina and cervix but not the uterus.

  - **Endocervical curettage** is useful for sampling the endocervix.

  - **D&C** is used to obtain a uterus sample.

  ☒ **Pregnant women** can undergo colposcopy and cervical biopsy, but not D&C.

Treatment:

- Imiquimod cream: used for genital warts and can be applied at home (3 times a week for 1 month).

- LEEP: used for high-grade carcinomas (CIN grade 2 and 3).

  - Complications: immediate complications are bleeding and infection. Long-term complications are cervical stenosis and cervical incompetence.

- For **pregnant** patients, use trichloroacetic acid.

- *Do not use podophyllin during **pregnancy**.

HPV vaccination: the first dose is administered at the age of 11–12 years, second dose (2 month later), and third dose (6 months) after the first dose.

Note: HPV vaccination can be given up to the age of 26 years **despite** previous sexual activity, previous HPV infection, or abnormal Pap smear.

Genital herpes simplex

HSV-2 is more likely to re-occur than HSV-1. Patients can transmit HSV-2 when asymptomatic and when **no** lesions are present. It is important to always use condoms with sexual partners even when lesions are not present. Condoms offers no protection when the lesion is not within the area covered by the condom (e.g. pubic area).

Treatment:

- Oral acyclovir 200 mg × 5/day for 7 days.
- If resistant to acyclovir, treat with foscarnet.

Note: Topical acyclovir is less effective, but can help alleviate pain.

Haemophilus ducreyi

More common in developing countries. Gram-negative coccobacillary organism that causes a disease known as **chancroid**, which results in genital lesion/s that begin as papules, vesicles, pustules, and develop into ulcers over 72 hours.

Hx/PE: These ulcers are **not** indurated and commonly have irregular borders. Lesions are very painful and often involve inguinal lymph nodes.

Diagnosis: Clinical diagnosis, PCR, or Gram stain culture (gram negative with a "school of fish" appearance).

Treatment: Single dose of IM Ceftriaxone and oral azithromycin.

Dysmenorrhea

Primary dysmenorrhea

Absence of pathology. Menstrual pain associated with ovulatory cycles. Excess PGF2α causes uterine vasoconstriction and sustained contraction.

Hx/PE: Pelvic pain usually "midline," pain can radiate to the back and inner thighs, occurs in the first few days before or during menstruation. Can be accompanied with headache, nausea, and vomiting.

Diagnosis: Rule out secondary dysmenorrhea. Order hCG levels, pelvic examination with cultures, and pelvic ultrasonography.

Treatment:

- First line: NSAIDs (anti-prostaglandin agents) and topical heat pads.
- Second line: OCPs (lighter and shorter periods).

Secondary dysmenorrhea

Menstrual pain caused by secondary pathology. Common causes are endometriosis, adenomyosis, fibroids, pelvic tumors, adhesions, and PID.

Hx/PE: Physical exam may include cervical motion tenderness, adnexal tenderness, cervical discharge, vaginal odor, or masses.

Diagnosis:

- First step: urine or serum hCG levels.
- Order: CBC, urinalysis, STD panel, stool guaiac, and pelvic ultrasonography.
- Rule out urinary, GI, and OBGYN causes.

Treatment: Treat underlying cause: STDs (antibiotics), fibroids and adenomyosis (OCPs), and masses (surgery may be necessary).

Endometriosis

Genetic predisposition plays a role and etiology is not completely clear. Endometrial glans and stroma **outside** the uterine cavity. Can cause infertility (50%), adhesions, and intestinal obstruction.

Hx/PE: Cyclical pelvic or rectal pain, dyspareunia, dysmenorrhea, and irregular periods.

Diagnosis:

- Serum hCG, pelvic examination, and pelvic ultrasonography.
- Definitive diagnosis is laparoscopy (lesion visualization) dark brown lesions, giving the uterus a "powder-burned" appearance; termed as "chocolate cysts" when present in the ovary. If not visualized biopsy uterus.

Treatment:

- First line: combination OCPs (regulates hormones).
- Second line: **pulsatile** GnRH agonist (leuprolide) and danazol.
- Next step: if medications are unsuccessful, laparoscopic lysis of adhesions can improve fertility.
- Definitive surgical treatment: TAH/BSO (in case of severe symptoms and when fertility is not desired).
- Patients who desire pregnancy can use clomiphene.

Note: **Danazol** (is progesterone-like, so has uterus protective action) can cause acne and hirsutism Can be used to treat endometriosis and fibrocystic breast cancer.

Adenomyosis

Benign lesions with presence of endometrial glands and stroma **within** the myometrium. Can be associated with C-section, pregnancy, endometriosis, and abortions.

Hx/PE: Non-cyclical pain, tender uterus, menorrhagia, dyspareunia, dysmenorrhea, and enlarged uterus.

Diagnosis: Serum hCG, pelvic examination, and transvaginal ultrasonography (enlarged **symmetric** uterus).

Treatment:

- NSAIDs, OCPs, pulsatile GnRH agonist (leuprolide), and danazol.
- Conservative surgical treatment: Endometrial ablation resection using hysteroscopy.
- Definitive: surgical hysterectomy.

Uterine leiomyomas

Benign lesions of the smooth muscle with growth of the myometrium. Large fibroids can cause obstruction of the colon and bladder (constipation and urinary retention). Risk of anemia and infertility.

Hx/PE: The majority are asymptomatic; **non-tender** uterus; dysmenorrhea, dyspareunia, and irregular heavy menstrual periods.

Diagnosis:

- Urine or serum hCG levels (rule out pregnancy) and CBC (rule out anemia).
- Transvaginal ultrasonography: uterine myomas are usually **asymmetric**.

Treatment:

- NSAIDs, OCPs, danazol, and GnRH analogs (decrease the size of the myomas).
- **Myomectomy** is the treatment of choice when conservative treatment is not successful and pregnancy is desired in future. Surgical treatment can also be considered in this case.
- If future pregnancy is not desired, consider hysterectomy.
- OCPs are controversial and not the treatment of choice for large fibroids.

Note: Often, patients do not need treatment; observation is sufficient for asymptomatic patients.

Ectopic pregnancy

Pregnancy outside the uterus with the most common location being the ampulla.

Hx/PE: **Triad**: abdominal pain, amenorrhea, and vaginal bleeding.

Diagnosis:

- First test for stable patients is serial hCG level testing (>1,500 IU/L), with observation of appropriate doubling in 48 hour.
- Transvaginal ultrasonography (more specific) **or** transabdominal ultrasonography (less specific). These tests help detect pregnancy outside of the uterus.
- Cross matching and Rh factor testing for mother.

Treatment:

- If **small** (<3.5cm) and unruptured, give MTX.
- If **larger** (>3.5cm), consider **salpingectomy** (if ruptured) or **salpingostomy** (if not ruptured). These procedures cause risk of future ectopic pregnancies.
- Tubal rupture (**obstetric emergency**), will need laparoscopy/ salpingectomy (removal of fallopian tube **plus** pregnancy).
- Give RhoGam to Rh-negative mother.

Pseudocyesis

Etiology is unknown but strong psychological influence is suggested. It is a relatively uncommon condition where females think they are pregnant but are not.

Hx/PE: Symptoms similar to a true pregnancy such as nausea, vomiting, abdominal distention (most common sign), absence of menses, and breast tenderness.

Diagnosis: hCG level (negative) and transvaginal ultrasonography (no intrauterine pregnancy).

Treatment: Psychotherapy and counseling.

Polycystic ovarian syndrome (Stein-Leventhal syndrome)

Common endocrine disorder in reproductive women. Increased LH stimulated by the theca cells increases the level of androgens, which in turn decrease the production of SHBG by the liver, leading to increased levels of free testosterone.

Hx/PE: Oligomenorrhea, mild acne, obesity, hirsutism, abnormal hair growth, glucose intolerance (highest risk), and infertility.

Diagnosis:

- Rule out causes of amenorrhea with hCG, prolactin, TSH, and FSH/LH ratio.
- Pelvic ultrasonography (first step) "pearl necklace sign" may be visible.
- Increased total testosterone and DHEAS levels.
- 17-OH progesterone and 24-hour urine free cortisol (to rule out CAH).
- Fasting glucose level (to rule out diabetes).
- Lipid panel (to rule out hyperlipidemia).

Treatment:

- First step to regain fertility is weight loss.
- Women who are **not** attempting to conceive can be treated with a combination OCPs and metformin.
- Women who are attempting to conceive can be treated with clomiphene +/- metformin.
- In cases of hirsutism, treat with OCPs (first line), spironolactone, and metformin.
- If patient develops pyelonephritis, treat with gentamycin and ampicillin.

Overall treatment:

- Weight loss, exercise, diet, glucose control (metformin), blood pressure (HTZC), and lipids (statins).

Complications: infertility, diabetes, hyperlipidemia, miscarriage, endometrial cancer, and breast cancer.

Infertility

Defined as the inability to conceive after 12 months of normal, regular, and unprotected sexual activity.

➤ Primary infertility: no prior pregnancy.

➤ Secondary infertility: has had prior pregnancy.

Diagnosis:

- In women, order hCG level (first test for women), TSH, and prolactin.
- In men, rule out infertility first with **semen analysis** which looks for semen pathology, followed by TSH, prolactin, and karyotype.
- **Ovulatory factors**: advanced age (menopause), abnormal TSH, abnormal prolactin, PCOS, and menstrual cycle abnormalities.
- **Tubal/pelvic factors**: PID, endometriosis, tubal surgery, and pelvic adhesions.

Treatment:

- Medication options: clomiphene citrate, pulsatile GnRH analog, FSH, and metformin.
- Hyperprolactinemia: cabergoline/bromocriptine.
- Hypothyroidism: levothyroxine.
- If medications fail, perform intrauterine insemination and in vitro fertilization.

Toxic shock syndrome (TSS)

Caused by *S. aureus* exotoxin (TSST-1) often within a week of menstrual period, caused by tampon use (more common with high absorptive tampons). Super antigen toxin activates T cells receptor binding with MHC II.

Hx/PE: Fever (102.0 F), low blood pressure, vomiting, confusion, and macular erythematous rash in palms and soles. Desquamation of rash in 10-14 days.

Diagnosis: CBC, ESR, electrolytes, blood culture, urinalysis, urine culture, and pelvic examination.

Treatment:

- Supportive treatment: ICU admission, hydration and/or vasopressors, if needed.
- There is **no** clear evidence of effective treatment with nafcillin, oxacillin (MSSA), or vancomycin (MRSA). Antibiotics can be administered as per the discretion of the medical practitioner.

Ovarian torsion
Medical emergency

Occurs when the ovary is completely twisted, thereby occluding blood supply. Can cause complications such as necrosis, infertility, infection, and sepsis.

Risk factors: ovarian cysts, ovarian tumors, and trauma.

Hx/PE: Severe acute unilateral adnexal pain.

Diagnosis:

- Cannot be made definitively without surgery.
- Immediate Doppler sonography.
- Order: serum hCG and pelvic ultrasonography.

Treatment: Laparoscopy surgery, first attempt to untwist ovary **oophoropexy**; then perform **oophorectomy**, if necrosis occurs.

Pelvic organ prolapse

Common after multiple vaginal births, advanced age, prior pelvic surgery, obesity, increased abdominal pressure, and chronic constipation.

Hx/PE: Bulging or protrusion of the vaginal tissue through the vagina, urinary or fecal incontinence, dyspareunia, and incomplete bladder emptying.

Diagnosis: Valsalva maneuver in lithotomy position.

Treatment:

- High-fiber diet (in case of constipation) and Kegel exercises.
- Weight reduction (in case of obesity).
- Limit straining and lifting, **vaginal pessaries** (temporarily) in women who do not want surgery.
- Surgery (definitive) with **vagina vault suspension**.

Note: Long-term use of pessaries can pose the risk of vaginal or cervical cancer.

Gynecological cancers

Endometrial cancer

Most common type of uterine cancer that arises from the endometrium and more common after menopause. Starts as atypical endometrial hyperplasia and develops into adenocarcinoma. Commonly caused by unopposed estrogen and obesity.

➤ **Type I**: common with metabolic syndrome and related to unopposed estrogen.

➤ **Type II**: no vaginal bleed and worse prognosis (more related to p53, rather than estrogen).

Hx/PE: Weight loss, fever, pelvic pain, vaginal discharge, and postcoital bleeding (usually >45 years of age).

Diagnosis:

- Vaginal ultrasonography (to measure endometrial thickness):
  - If **less** than 4 mm, favorable prognosis.
  - If **greater** than 4 mm, endocervical/endometrial biopsy needed.

- Dilation and curettage: biopsy endometrial tissue.
- In case of adenocarcinoma, do a metastatic work-up.

Treatment:
- Treatment options are surgery (TAH/BSO), radiation, and chemotherapy.
- Use of prostaglandins are protective.

Screening is not recommended unless bleeding is observed in postmenopausal women.

Note: Tamoxifen use can increase risk of endometrial cancer.

Cervical cancer

Average age of diagnosis is 45 years with common risk factors being early onset of sexual intercourse, multiple sexual partners, and smoking history.

➤ Cancer in the upper 1/3rd of the **cervix**, is usually an adenoma.

➤ Cancer in the lower 2/3rd of the **cervix**, is usually squamous cell cancer (most common).

➤ The squamocolumnar junction is located in the ectocervix.

➤ HPV is found in almost all cervical cancers (commonly HPV 16 and 18).

➤ HPV 16 more commonly causes squamous cell carcinoma.

➤ HPV 18 commonly causes adenocarcinoma.

Staging:
- Stage 0 (carcinoma in situ).
- Stage I (confined to the cervix).
- Stage II (beyond the cervix not in the pelvic wall or lower 1/3rd of the vagina).
- Stage III (disease in the pelvic wall or lower 1/3rd of the vagina).
- Stage IV (invades bladder or rectum).

Classifications:

- **CIN I**: mild dysplasia.
- **CIN II**: moderate dysplasia.
- **CIN III**: severe dysplasia.
- **Invasive cancer**: this is real cancer.

Hx/PE: Postcoital spotting, cervical ulceration, metrorrhagia, and malodorous non-pruritic discharge.

Diagnosis:

- Two Pap smears are needed to confirm ASCUS, with repeat Pap smear in 3–6 months after the first abnormal Pap. Order cytology **plus** HPV DNA typing.
  - In case of positive HPV DNA typing for HPV 16 or 18, colposcopy and ectocervical biopsy will be required.
  - If the second Pap smear result is negative, 2 consecutive Pap smears will be needed to confirm negative ASCUS.
- Endocervical curettage: all **non-pregnant** patients who undergo a colposcopy and ectocervical biopsy will need to undergo endocervical curettage.
- **Pregnant** women will have the same work-up as non-pregnant women with the exception of endocervical curettage.

Treatment:

- Is based on biopsy; treatment is very complicated and patients are referred to the oncology team.
- If CIN II or CIN III, then LEEP is the treatment of choice. Other options are cold knife conization, cryotherapy, and CO_2 laser.
- Consider radiation and chemotherapy in young females and patients who desire children.
- Radical hysterectomy can be curative in localized cancer (might be a good option in elderly patients).
- **Pregnancy**: if ASCUS is found on Pap smear, then repeat Pap smear (in 3-6 months), order cytology, and HPV DNA testing. If HPV testing is positive for aggressive genotypes or second Pap smears demonstrates ASCUS, then colposcopy and ectocervical biopsy are required.
- **Pregnancy**:

- In cases of **invasive cancer** and less than 24 weeks of pregnancy, perform hysterectomy or radiation therapy.
- In cases of **invasive cancer** and greater than 24 weeks of pregnancy, provide conservative management up to 32 weeks with cesarean delivery and definitive treatment.

Screening:

- Do not screen women younger than 21 years of age (strong recommendation). Unless history of HIV, SLE, or immunocompromised.
- Start screening women at the age of 21 despite age of first vaginal intercourse (strong recommendation).
- From age 21–29 years, screen every 2–3 years using liquid-based cervical cytology **only** (if normal Pap smear results are obtained).
- If the patient is aged >30 years and has had three previous normal Pap smear results, then screen every 5 years with cytology **plus** HPV testing.
- Can stop screening after 65 years (if three normal Pap smears or no strong risk factors).

Fun facts:

- Conduct colposcopy and ectocervical biopsy, if malignant type HPV is detected.
- Colposcopy and ectocervical biopsy can be done in pregnant women.
- If colposcopy and ectocervical biopsy results are unsatisfactory, perform endocervical curettage (if not pregnant).
- Malignant work-up would include **cystoscopy** (rule out bladder metastasis) and **proctoscopy** (colon metastasis).

Note: Breast cancer screening should be stopped at 75 years and cervical cancer screening should be stopped after 65 years.

Vulvar cancer

Almost 90% are squamous lesions and occur in women aged >50 years of age, more commonly on the labia majora. Risk factors are similar to those of cervical cancer: HPV infection (HPV 16, 18, and 31), multiple sexual partners, cervical cancer, and smoking.

Hx/PE: Vulvar pruritus, localized pain, irritation, and ulcerations with raised thickened nodular type lesions.

Diagnosis:

- Requires a vulvar punch biopsy:
    - VIN I (mild dysplasia)
    - VIN II (moderate dysplasia).
    - VIN III (sever form including, carcinoma in situ).

Treatment:

- **High-grade VIN**:
    - Can range from laser ablation, simple vulvectomy, wide local excision, to topical chemotherapy.
- **If invasive**:
    - Radical vulvectomy and regional lymphadenectomy **or** wide local excision with inguinal lymph node dissection, +/- chemotherapy and radiation.

Vaginal cancer

Cancer occurring in the vagina more commonly caused by squamous cell carcinoma or adenocarcinoma (less common; clear cell adenocarcinoma), usually in postmenopausal women.

Risk factors: Long-term pessary use, prolapse, low socioeconomic status, radiation from cervical cancer, multiple sexual partners, and DES exposure.

Hx/PE: Abnormal vaginal bleeding, abnormal discharge, postcoital bleeding, and dyspareunia.

Diagnosis: Pap smear, cytology, colposcopy, and biopsy.

Treatment:

- Consider local excision, if small.
- Partial or complete **vaginectomy** (if large or increased staging).
- Invasive disease: radiation therapy.

Note: Squamous cell carcinoma in the lower part of the vagina is often treated with radiation therapy alone.

Ovarian tumors

Most common gynecological tumor leading to death (early disease is rarely detected). The tumors are commonly epithelial in origin with a bimodal distribution. Terminal illness is defined as death within 6 months.

- ➤ **Germ cell tumors**: common in children and elevation of markers will depend on tumor type (LAD, βHCG, or AFP).
- ➤ **Epithelial tumors**: common in elderly patients with elevated CA-125 and CEA levels.
- ➤ **Granulosa-Theca**: endometrial hyperplasia caused by estrogen secretion.
- ➤ **Sertoli-Leydig cell**: masculinization caused by testosterone secretion.
- ➤ **Dermoid cysts**: benign tumors with all 3 germ layers.

Risks: Bimodal age distribution (advanced age or young age), low parity, delayed childbirth, early menarche, late menopause, fertility medication, smoking, family history, Lynch II syndrome or hereditary nonpolyposis colorectal cancer, BRCA-1 mutation (more risk), and BRCA-2 (less risk).

Hx/PE: Usually asymptomatic in early stages; patients later present with mild GI symptoms or pelvic pressure and pain. Patients later present with abdominal distension, ascites, and adnexal mass.

Note: Breastfeeding and OCPs use for at least 5 years decreases the risk.

Diagnosis:

- First step is transvaginal or transabdominal ultrasonography.
- Tumor markers:
  - In **younger** patients, check LDH, AFP, and βHCG levels.
  - In **elderly** patients, check CA-125 and CEA levels, which are often associated with epithelial cancer.

- - **Pre**menopausal women with elevated CA-125 usually have benign disease.
  - **Post**menopausal women with elevated CA-125 usually have malignant disease.
- If Sertoli-Leydig tumor is suspected, check testosterone levels.
- If granulosa-theca tumor is suspected, check estrogen levels.
- If ascites measure serum-ascites albumin gradient.
- Biopsy via laparoscopy to determine benign vs malignant.

Screening is not usually recommended unless strong family history. In cases of strong family history, screen with CA-125 and transvaginal ultrasonography.

Treatment:

- Surgical options including unilateral or bilateral removal of ovaries (oophorectomy), the Fallopian tubes (salpingectomy), the uterus (hysterectomy), and the omentum (omentectomy).
  - **Premenarchal women**:
    - Mass measuring >2 cm requires exploratory laparotomy.
  - **Premenopausal women**:
    - Mass measuring <8 cm, mobile, and unilateral, observe for 4 to 6 weeks.
    - Mass measuring >8 cm or unchanging mass, surgical evaluation needed.
  - **Postmenopausal women:**
    - If asymptomatic, unilateral simple cysts <5 cm, follow with ultrasonography and CA-125.
    - If palpable or >5 cm, exploratory laparotomy required.
  - **Premenopausal** patient, consider salpingo-oophorectomy.
  - **Postmenopausal** patient, consider TAH-SBO and chemotherapy.

Note:

✓Debulking surgery with para-aortic nodal and pelvic nodal

sampling, followed by chemotherapy (cisplatin and paclitaxel) is the best treatment for advanced stages of cancer or metastatic disease.

✓ Patients with ovarian cancer are at a risk of ovarian torsion.

Breast pathology

Acute mastitis

Inflammation of the breast tissue caused by milk stasis **or** oral flora of the baby (S. aureus). Seen almost exclusively in breastfeeding women during first few months postpartum.

Risk factors: infant with inappropriate attachment, long periods between feedings, decreased feedings, and tight clothing or bras.

Hx/PE: Present with breast erythema, tenderness, mild fever, and possible breast engorgement.

Diagnosis:
- Mainly a clinical diagnosis unless suspicion of breast cancer, which will warrant a work-up.
- Can consider fluid culture and breast ultrasonography.

Treatment:
- Milk drainage helps remove blockage or infection; encouraged to feed newborn from affected breast.
- Underlying infection can treat with penicillin antibiotics (dicloxacillin) or azithromycin, if allergic to penicillin.
- First-generation cephalosporin (cephalexin).

Note: Do not give doxycycline while breastfeeding.

Fibroadenoma

Slow growing benign breast tumor which is the most common breast lesion in women aged <30 years. **Cystosarcoma phyllodes**, usually benign and can grow to larger sizes (is basically, a large fibroadenoma).

Hx/PE: Round, rubbery, mobile, non-tender mass, usually solitary, and size does not change during menstrual period.

Diagnosis:
- First step: Breast examination.
- Breast ultrasonography (cystic vs. solid mass).
- FNA or needle biopsy (rarely needed).
- Excision of lesion, if unsure of pathology.
- Cystosarcoma phyllodes: May require surgical removal.

Treatment: Observation or excision (if size > 2–4 cm).

Fibrocystic disease

Common benign breast condition; which responds to hormonal changes and is usually observed in the childbearing age and rarely found in postmenopausal woman. Can be associated with trauma and caffeine.

Hx/PE: Cyclical mastalgia and swelling just before menstruation. Breast lesion with rapid fluctuation in size and lumpy consistency "oatmeal with raisins."

Diagnosis:
- First step is breast examination.
- Second step: Breast ultrasonography can show simple cyst or complex cyst.
  - **Simple cyst**: conduct FNA.
  - **Complex cyst**: conduct core biopsy.
- Mammography may have limited use in younger females.
- High suspicion of fibrocystic disease, follow-up a week **after** the next menstrual period to check if the tumor has shrunk.
- FNA is helpful in distinguishing pathology.
  - If cyst resolves after FNA more likely fibrocystic disease.
- FNA shows blood **or** does not go away, then core biopsy is recommended.

Note:

- ✓ If mass goes away after FNA (takes about a week); **no** more tests needed.

- ✓ Each time the cyst grows, repeat breast ultrasonography and FNA, which should regress the cysts.

- ✓ On the third recurrence, the patient will need excisional biopsy, and malignancy will need to be ruled out.

Treatment:

- Decrease caffeine, administer danazol (helps relieve severe pain, but can cause acne and hirsutism).

- OCPs (controversial) can also help control hormonal levels.

Note: After the cyst has regressed with FNA, It is important to schedule a follow-up in a month with a breast ultrasonography.

Types of breast cancers

➤ **Inflammatory breast carcinoma**: erythema, edema, warm, pitting, peau d'orange "orange peel," appearance, and ulcerations. Difficult to diagnosis, as does not present with breast lumps. Prognosis is poor.

➤ **Paget's breast disease**: usually cancer overlies the area of the nipple. Can coexist with DCIS or invasive carcinoma. Look for "eczematous", scaling, inverted nipple, or ulcerated lesion involving the areolar area.

➤ **Ductal carcinoma in situ (DCIS)**: developing from the breast ducts. Is a type of pre-cancerous or non-invasive cancerous classified as stage 0. Usually found on mammography screening. Observation or surgical removal with or without radiation and tamoxifen.

➤ **Lobular carcinoma in situ (LCIS)**: developing from the lobules. Is a type of pre-cancerous or non-invasive cancerous classified as stage 0. Usually found on mammography screening. Usually treatment is conservative with close follow-up.

➤ **Invasive ductal carcinoma**: most common breast cancer.

Breast cancer

Most common invasive cancer in women and the second most common cause of death. Occurs most commonly in the upper left quadrant.

Risk factors: female gender, advanced age, first-degree relative, BRCA-1, BRCA-2, high-fat, low-fiber diet, excessive alcohol consumption, HRT, obesity, first full-term pregnancy after age of 35 years, early menarche, and late menopause.

Hx/PE:

➤ **Early findings:** asymptomatic, single nodule, non-tender, firm, and ill-defined margins.

➤ **Later findings:** possible breast enlargement, erythemia, edema, pain, and skin or nipple retraction.

➤ Be aware of supraclavicular lymphadenopathy and edema of the arm.

Diagnosis:

- First step in **pre**menopausal women if <30 years of age is breast ultrasonography (solid vs. cyst). If solid cyst then consider mammography despite its lack of specificity in women <30 years of age.

- If positive findings on ultrasonography or mammography, next step is core biopsy.

- First step in **post**menopausal women is always mammography.

- If positive biopsy results, obtain receptor status (estrogen receptor, progesterone receptor, and HER2/neu status).

- Tumor marker: CA 15-3, CA 27-29, or CEA.

- Metastatic disease to the bone can demonstrate elevated alkaline phosphatase levels.

- Pregnant women can undergo mammography (safe during pregnancy) and core biopsy.

- BRCA genetic testing is not a routine screening test but can be used for screening in cases of family history of breast cancer and ovarian cancer.

Treatment:

- Hormone-receptor positive and **pre**menopausal, administer **tamoxifen**.

- Hormone-receptor positive and **post**menopausal, administer **anastrozole**.
- **HER2/neu**-positive, use **trastuzumab**.
- Hormone-receptor negative, patient should receive chemotherapy and radiation.
- Radiation can be given by external beam radiotherapy or internal radiotherapy (brachytherapy).
- Surgery:
  - Perform a lumpectomy plus axillary node sampling, If tumor <4 cm.
  - Perform a mastectomy plus axillary node sampling, If tumor >4 cm.

Fun facts:
- Negative FNA does not rule out breast cancer in a middle-aged female and would need a core biopsy (larger sample) for further examination.
- FNA can be helpful for fibroadenoma and fibrocystic disease.
- Mammogram is not as specific in young females (increased connective tissue) or pregnancy (increased breast milk). However, there is no harm in attempting.
- **Radical mastectomy** is no longer done (it involves removing the pectorals muscles in addition to breast tissue).
- Mastectomy alone might be helpful for palliative care.
- During pregnancy can perform mastectomy or lumpectomy.
  - Radiation therapy is contraindicated at **any** time during pregnancy, and chemotherapy is contraindicated in the first trimester.
  - No need to terminate pregnancy.
- Can use tamoxifen as a breast cancer prophylaxis:
  - Used in high-risk women with positive estrogen and progesterone receptors.
- TNM staging is the most reliable indicator of prognosis.
  - Poor prognosis in case of lymph node involvement.
  - Good prognosis if estrogen and progesterone-receptor positive.

- Breast and prostate are more likely to metastasize to the bone than other cancers (measure alkaline phosphate levels).
- Conservative lumpectomy is contraindicated:
  - In cases of large tumor.
  - Subareolar location.
  - Multifocal tumors.
  - Fixation to the chest wall.
  - Involves the nipple or overlying skin.
- Tamoxifen can increase risk of endometrial cancer and DVTs.
- Trastuzumab: related to cardiotoxicity which is reversible once discontinuation.
- Nonbloody nipple discharge more likely to be **intraductal papilloma**.
- If bloody discharge, more likely to be a malignant condition.

Breast cancer medications

Tamoxifen

<u>Mechanism of action</u>: *selective estrogen receptor modulator* (SERM).

<u>Use:</u> breast cancer in **pre**menopausal women (if positive estrogen and progesterone receptors); helps increase bone density (reduce risk of osteoporosis) and decreases cardiovascular mortality.

<u>Side effects</u>: endometrial cancer and thromboembolism (strokes, MI, and DVTs).

<u>Screening</u>: need to screen with annual pap smears, while on medication.

Raloxifene

<u>Mechanism of action:</u> SERM.

<u>Use</u>: is approved for postmenopausal osteoporosis and breast cancer patients.

Side effects:

- Increased risk of endometrial cancer and DVTs.
- Exacerbation of hot flashes and menopausal symptoms.

Contraindicated for patients with thromboembolic disease.

Note: stop medication about 1 month before surgery because of risk of thrombosis.

Anastrozole

Mechanism of action: *Aromatase inhibitor.*

Use: approved for breast cancer in post-menopausal women who have hormone-receptor positive cancer. Can use in patients with risk of DVTs.

Side effect: leads to osteoporosis but not DVTs.

Breast augmentation

Breast implants

Most common complications are local capsular contracture that can cause local pain.

➤ Breast implants do not cause autoimmune disease.
➤ There is no risk of breastfeeding or pregnancy complications.
➤ Keep in mind that women should have normal scheduled breast examinations.

Index

Index, cont'd

Index, cont'd

secondary amenorrhea 60
secondary dysmenorrhea 72
secondary infertility 77
septic pelvic thrombophlebitis 42
Sertoli-Leydig cell 84
Sheehan's syndrome 48
sodium citrate 47
Stein-Leventhal syndrome 76
sterile speculum examination 23
stillbirth 22

T

tamoxifen 89, 91
the implant 65
the ring 65
toxic shock syndrome 77
transdermal contraceptive patch 64
trastuzumab 90
trichomoniasis 68
Turner syndrome 59
Tzanck smear 11

U

Ulipristal 19
umbilical cord prolapse 37
uterine atony 48
uterine leiomyomas 74

V

vaginal atrophy 62
vaginal cancer 83
vaginal pessaries 79
vaginal yeast infection 67
vagina vault suspension 79
Valsalva maneuver 79
vasa previa 35
vasectomy 66
venlafaxine 63
vulvar cancer 82

www.ingramcontent.com/pod-product-compliance
Lightning Source LLC
Chambersburg PA
CBHW040826180526
45159CB00001B/89